Enabling Relationships in Health and Social Care

For Butterworth-Heinemann:

Senior commissioning editor: Heidi Allen
Development editor: Robert Edwards
Project manager: Morven Dean
Designer: George Ajayi

Enabling Relationships in Health and Social Care

A Guide for Therapists

By

John Swain BSc, PGCE, MSc, PhD

Professor of Disability and Inclusion, Northumbria University, Newcastle upon Tyne, UK

Jim Clark MA, Cert Ed, Ad Dip Drama, Ad Dip Spec Ed

Head of Division, Health, Community and Education Studies, Northumbria University, Newcastle upon Tyne, UK

Sally French BSc, MSc (Psych), MSc (Soc), MSCP Dip TP PhD

Senior Lecturer, Department of Allied Health Professions, University of Hertfordshire, Hatfield, UK

Karen Parry BEd PhD

Inter Agency Development Officer, Sunderland City Council, Tyne and Wear, UK

Frances Reynolds BSc, Dip Psych Couns, PhD

Senior Lecturer in Psychology, Department of Health and Social Care, Brunel University, Middlesex, UK

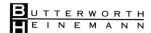

OXFORD   AUCKLAND   BOSTON   JOHANNESBURG   MELBOURNE   NEW DELHI   2004

BUTTERWORTH-HEINEMANN
An imprint of Elsevier Limited

ISBN 0 7506 5274 8

British Library Cataloguing in Publication Data
A catalogue record for this book is available from the British Library

Library of Congress Cataloging in Publication Data
A catalog record for this book is available from the Library of Congress

Note
Medical knowledge is constantly changing. As new information becomes available, changes in treatment, procedures, equipment and the use of drugs become necessary. The authors and the publishers have taken care to ensure that the information given in this text is accurate and up to date. However, readers are strongly advised to confirm that the information, especially with regard to drug usage, complies with the latest legislation and standards of practice.

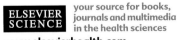

your source for books,
journals and multimedia
in the health sciences

www.elsevierhealth.com

Printed in China

The
publisher's
policy is to use
paper manufactured
from sustainable fores

Contents

Stumbling on: an introduction
John Swain

WHAT IS THIS BOOK ABOUT?

In the early 1990s I wrote a book that came to be entitled *The use of counselling skills: a guide for therapists* (Swain 1995). It was published in the Skills for Practice series edited by Sally French and Jo Laing. Though it may not have revolutionized therapy practice, it was well received and sold well enough for the question of a second edition to arise, and with it something of a dilemma. Was it simply a matter of updating the existing text or was it time to begin afresh? Deliberations with the publisher led to a compromise: yes, it was possible to publish a book that follows on from and can be considered a second edition of *The use of counselling skills*; but also a book that is sufficiently distinctive to be a new text and merit a new title.

This introduction sets the scene for the book as a whole, mapping the path from the original text to our present endeavour. It is not, however, an easily defined route. Whilst generally reading around I came (stumbled) across Potter's thoughts on 'stumbling'. He seemed to encapsulate the ethos of this introductory chapter:

> *Stumbling* is wonderful, with its aura of happenstance and unintentionality; it is surely no accident that 'stumbling over' is both a description of an action/behaviour and a more idiomatic gloss on finding something by chance. Such things are often *precisely* what is at issue in practical situations . . . (1998, p. 34)

The terrain around which I am stumbling is certainly similar to that of the previous book. It is about people, their feelings, thoughts and desires. It is also about those subtle and complex processes that connect people: communications, awareness of themselves and others, and personal relationships. This is, however, a different book with a different title. So what has changed? My first answer would be that I have changed and I would want to say, 'I am not the person I was'. In fact, I am not even sure I ever was the person I was. The phrase 'I am not the person I was' is based on the conception of the self as an entity, which was a definable, knowable reality and is now a different definable, knowable reality. I am by no means alone in such reflections on changing understandings of self or social identity. Indeed, as Jenkins (1996) suggests, the centrality of 'social identity' as 'one of the unifying frameworks of intellectual debate in the 1990s' is possibly a sign of the times. Echoing a widely held belief that 'the times' are themselves rapidly changing, Jenkins writes:

> Popular concern about identity is, in large part perhaps, a reflection of the uncertainty produced by rapid change and cultural contact: our social maps no longer fit our social landscapes. (1996, p. 9)

In the changing social maps there is an erosion of the dichotomies of self–society and self–other, and the emergence of the notion of 'relational selves'. For me this can be crystalized by re-writing the well known Cartesian phrase, 'I think, therefore I am', to 'I relate, therefore I am'. Gergen is more expansive:

> . . . the conception of relational being reduces the debilitating gap between self and other, the sense of oneself as alone and the other as alien and untrustworthy. Whatever we are, from the present standpoint, is either directly or indirectly with others. . . . We are made up of each other. . . . we are mutually constituting. (1999, pp. 137–138)

In the previous book I focused on 'counselling skills', albeit in a broad framework; that is, the de-contextualized behaviours of individual therapists. In this book we shift the emphasis to therapists as relational beings and the central focus to relationships between people, rather than the skills that one person might use on another. It is written around the idea that health and social care can be enabling. The phrase 'enabling relationships' in the title has two related meanings. It refers to the processes of enabling, or enhancing, relationships between participants: professionals and clients. It also invokes the power of relationships to change people and construct change. Professional support is an essentially human activity that needs to be under-stood in terms of the relationships, the dynamics of communication and the people involved. Empowerment has meaning within the broader historical and social context of human relations and of hierarchical power structures within our society. The subject of this book is the empowerment of clients through professional support in emancipation from discrimination and oppression.

The language we use is particularly potent in framing thinking and reflection. I have already introduced many terms that are obscure, and need unpacking and questioning. What is 'empowerment', 'emancipation', 'power' and 'oppression'? This is not simply a matter of definition. Words do, that is, they have social significance, as well as meaning. From the outset, the labelling of people in the context of this book bears particular significance. What is the significance of the use of the term 'professional'? I, along with many other people, could claim to have done activities with my children that could be called physiotherapy, occupational therapy, speech and language therapy, counselling, social work and teaching – but not as a professional (or a multi-professional!). So what is the difference? The term 'client' is perhaps even more problematic as there are many alternatives: patient, service user and all the other labels that can be attached to people who receive therapy – autistic, aphasic, visually impaired, learning disabled and so on. We have chosen to use the term client(s), as this does not necessarily have medical connotations and can denote active agency rather than passivity.

The overall intention is to support therapists in constructing open and non-hierarchical relationships for shared decision-making, effective working part-nerships and mutual empowerment. In working towards this, the book offers a basis for a deepening understanding of human relations in the practice of therapy and reflection on practice within this context. This study of enabling relationships aims to help professionals to reflect on:

- themselves and others in terms of their relationships and the dynamics of communication
- professional support in processes of empowering clients to understand themselves better, and be more effective in defining and solving their own problems
- processes of empowerment in terms of emancipation from the barriers of institutional discrimination
- reflective practice in the development of enabling relationships.

We return to this key concept of reflection below.

WHO HAS WRITTEN THIS BOOK?

Another major change is that this book has five co-authors, rather than a single author. As an author, Mairian Corker (now Scott-Hill) (1994) asks herself 'who am I?' and in her 1994 publication quotes Foucault:

> Someone who is a writer is not simply doing his (sic) work in books, in what he publishes . . . his major work is, in the end, himself in the process of writing his books . . . the work includes the whole life as well as the text. The work is more than the work; the subject who is writing is part of the work. (1994, p. 184)

This is true for us. This book reflects our beliefs, feelings, intuitions and understanding which have developed over many years, and which we have had to confront and review as we write, and thus continue to develop. The very subject matter is not just academic or professional, but is personal, and political in the sense that the personal is political. It is for this reason that each chapter has a named author who can address you, the reader, as 'I', the writer. In writing this book we have attempted to be consistent in our approach, but allowed each of our separate voices to be expressed.

Returning to the quotation from Foucault, it is limited in conveying our experiences as authors. First, he writes as the sole author, whereas we write as five co-authors writing collaboratively. This book is, in a sense, the product and process of enabling relationships. Second, he does not mention the reader or the fact that he writes in relation to the reader. This book is in a very real sense produced by you, the reader, as much as it is by us, the authors, and below we shall begin to look at how the book might be used.

WHO IS THIS BOOK FOR?

It is for physiotherapists, occupational therapists, and speech and language therapists, as well as students of these professions. The topic, enabling relationships, is equally relevant to the three professions. This book is also intended for professional and non-professional educators and trainers in the therapy field. It can be argued that enabling relationships are important for all those who work in the human services, in either a formal or informal capacity. Professionals may be effective in the particular expertise of their own profession and still be deficient in terms of the human encounters involved. This book is, in general terms, relevant to a wide audience, though the particular examples and discussions are geared to therapists in health care.

HOW TO USE THIS BOOK

This book is about changing therapy practice through enabling relationships. It engages us in reviewing or reflecting on practice as a foundation for developing new possibilities, conceiving alternatives. It has, therefore, been designed as a book to be worked through as well as simply read. At various points within each chapter you will find **REFLECTIONS**. These are suggestions for 'exercises and activities' that are aimed at helping you get the most out of the ideas being discussed. The approach is based on the belief that there is no single certain way of engaging with the topic of enabling relationships. There are a number of processes that can be effective and can be drawn on in facilitating relational reflections. The first, of course, in a book entitled *Enabling Relationships*, is to work with others through the book. This might be a single partner, possibly a colleague, with whom you can engage in the 'reflections', or a series of partners with whom to engage as relevant throughout the book. For us, writing is a collaborative, relational activity, and we are suggesting that reading might be the same for you. This is by no means a novel suggestion (sorry about the pun). We learn to read as a shared activity and there are numerous 'book circles' within which reading is a joint, relational activity.

We learn about relationships through and within relationships. Furthermore, reflective practice is a collaborative activity: basically, professionals can learn more if they share their learning experiences with others. The more knowledge and experience is pooled, the richer will be the process of learning about human relations. Such collaboration incorporates both one-to-one and group situations.

Collaboration requires the establishment of trust in which people can communicate openly and freely. This involves discussion and negotiation around some complex issues relating to ethics and the processes of communication. For instance, there are questions of anonymity and confidentiality to be dealt with in an agreed code of ethics that might remain informal but is continually reviewed. Other issues include the invasion of privacy, the right to opt out and the establishment of equality in participation so that the group or one-to-one situation is not dominated or manipulated from one side.

REFLECTIONS

If it is possible, approach someone to be your partner as you work through the text and exercises. This may be a colleague, fellow student, client, or even someone not involved in therapy. Your partner will provide a sounding-board for you, particularly if you can work through the **REFLECTIONS** together. The partnership will also provide a focus for you when thinking about the qualities of relationships and communication. This book has been written so that you can work through it on your own, but from the stance taken within the book we would suggest that enabling relationships are best studied within enabling relationships.

In general terms, there are a number of principles behind this idea of reflective practice:

- The therapist wants to and can improve the processes of enabling relationships and the dynamics of communication in therapy.
- The therapist can take responsibility for the development of enabling relationships.
- Development requires the therapist to enquire into his or her own 'personal action theories' and practice in terms of the empowerment of clients and anti-discrimination.
- The processes of reflection are facilitated through collaboration with others.

The approach builds on notions of the 'reflective practitioner', summarized by Schön as follows:

> ... both ordinary people and professional practitioners often think about what they are doing, sometimes even while doing it ... It is this entire process of reflection-in-action which is central to the 'art' by which practitioners deal well with situations of uncertainty, instability, uniqueness and value conflict. (1983, p. 50)

Schön's work is widely referred to and drawn on by practitioners working in many different contexts.

Wilkinson (1988) suggests three distinct but interrelated forms of reflexivity: personal, functional and disciplinary. Although the original focus was research in the social sciences, Wilkinson provides a useful framework for reflecting on interpersonal relationships in therapy practice. *Personal reflexivity* requires the therapist to examine her or his individuality and its effects on therapy. This is the attempt to recognize and examine the motivations, interests, attitudes, values and beliefs that the therapist brings into therapy practice. *Functional reflexivity* relates to the therapist's role and the effect this may have on the process of therapy. The focus shifts to the interactions between therapists and clients, particularly the distribution of power within the therapy process, and the factors that shape the therapy process. These factors can include the structural elements of a profession: responsibilities and expectations, lines of authority and management, and so on. Professional bodies and codes of ethics or rules of conduct can have a bearing, as can state legislation. Finally, *disciplinary reflexivity* entails a critical stance towards therapy practice within broader debates about theory in relation to practice.

Thompson (2000, p.1) writes that practice informed by theory is necessary to:

- do justice to the complexity of the situations human service workers so frequently encounter
- avoid assumptions, prejudices and stereotypes that can lead to discrimination and oppression
- lay the foundations for a *developmental* approach, one which permits and facilitates continuous personal and professional development
- ensure a high level of motivation, challenge and commitment.

A common approach to reflexive practice is to keep a journal that documents your thoughts, feelings and experiences before, during and after therapy encounters. A journal is a written narrative, or story, of you, your relationships and the dynamics of your communication, and the ways in which you develop enabling relationships. This reflexive account concerns the reasoning for certain decisions and choices, changing directions and personal reactions. It can provide a resource for personal, functional and disciplinary reflection.

This book, then, is about 'stumbling on' together through reflecting on relationships and communication in practice. In developing understanding and challenging taken-for-granted assumptions, we look towards the broader historical and social context of therapy practice and possibilities for change. Overall, we hope that you find this book useful in empowering you in enabling relationships.

PART 1

In context

Working together can change things and can enable people to change things. Relationships are powerful, and, of course, if relationships can be enabling then they can also be disabling. Relationships can create change and can also maintain status quo. In Part 1 we explore the broad context of health and social care in therapy practice. The chapters set the scene for addressing enabling relationships. Relationships are fashioned between people in their interactions, understandings, purposes and desires. Relationships are also contained, restrained, shaped, limited, given meaning and also empowered within the broader social and historical context that people bring and that brings people to relationships. Part 1 is about stepping outside therapy practice to reflect on the personal and social worlds, the organizational contexts of health and social care, and the ethical decision-making within which therapists and clients engage in the provision of health and social care. In Chapter 1, John Swain looks at the personal and social worlds that both therapists and clients bring to therapy practice. So what's the story? He looks first at notions of self in the shifting sands of the rapidly changing social world, and ways of understanding ourselves and others as relational beings. The discussion then moves into the complexities of communication and, particularly, the dynamics of sharing meaning. He then looks into the broader context of social divisions and power relations – and the multiplicity of identities that we construct between us and within which we are constructed (such as man/woman, deaf/hearing, old/young, gay/straight). Frances Reynolds analyzes the organizational or systematic context of the relationships in therapy. She centrally focuses on partnerships as enabling relationships. Frances examines the conceptual and organizational barriers to genuine partnerships and possible strategies for overcoming them. Sally French turns to the involvement of therapists in people's lives, the values that therapists bring to their work and the processes of ethical decision-making therapy inevitably involves. Using examples from therapy practice, she explores the inherent complexities of ethics, showing how ethical issues pervade every aspect of therapy.

Chapter 1

What's the story?

John Swain

I approach this opening chapter, which is about stories of personal and social worlds, with some trepidation. It has a feeling of ultimate questions – who am I? What is the meaning of life? It is not, however, about ultimate answers, but rather taking a critical reflective stance to try to get behind what can seem common-sense answers. So rather than the meaning of life the chapter is more about 'Life, Jim, but not as we know it', to use a phrase associated with the television programme *Star Trek*. In more formal terms this is a process of deconstruction:

> The exploration or unravelling of the often 'hidden' internal contradictions, assumptions and repressed meanings of a text, discourse or practice. By revealing these repressed meanings, deconstructive analyses function to destabilize, subvert and resist dominant forms of knowledge. (Nightingale & Cromby 1999, pp. 225–226)

This critically reflective stance will run throughout this book, a theme that drives our discussions. We hope that as you work through the book this will be a basis for action and change. As McLeod states:

> Often the first steps in initiating change involve not direct action but creating a framework for understanding what is happening, and how things might be different. (1998, p. 256)

A quotation from Martin Luther King Jr provides a good example of critical reflection that is as relevant today as it was in the 1960s:

> Today, psychologists have a favourite word, and that word is maladjusted. I tell you there are some things in our social system to which I am proud to be maladjusted. I shall never be adjusted to lynch mobs, segregation, economic inequalities, 'the madness of militarism', and self-defeating physical violence. The salvation of the world lies in the maladjusted. (Freedman & Combs 1996, p. 59)

There are many different ways of looking at therapy and all it may encompass, including the diverse range of problems that are faced, from every side, and the whole gamut of activities in which therapists engage. We are exploring, in particular, therapy as support, in all its different forms, and the human relations of support. From this vantage point, therapy is not regarded as a set of techniques, largely medical in orientation, that can be brought to bear on a set of problems, themselves largely medical in manifestation. Rather, therapy is seen as an essentially human activity that needs to be understood in terms of the people involved, their relationships, processes of communication and the broader social and historical context in which 'I', 'you and I' and 'we' are understood.

This exploration of enabling relationships begins by examining the key concepts that provide the compass points for navigating the implications of enabling relationships in therapy practice. These are understandings of self and/or identity, processes of relating and communication between people, and the social relations of power in society.

I: UNDERSTANDING SELF

The concept of self and the transformation of its meaning has provoked debate within philosophy and the social sciences for 'two millennia' (Bruner 1995, p. 25). The common-sense view in contemporary Western societies is that each of us is an entity, a 'self' or 'I', irrespective of the context or the society in which we live. The concept of 'personality' is associated with this view – personality conceived in terms of traits or characteristics and causing behaviour. To be successful at sport, for instance, can be thought to require a competitive streak, and an introverted person will not be the life and soul of a party. As Gough & McFadden point out (2001, p. 74) there are parallels between such informal theories of self and more formal theories within the psychology literature, particularly personality theories. Theories can assume that personality is:

- identifiable (and measurable)
- stable over time (i.e. fixed)
- internal consistency (all characteristics fit together)
- the (main) cause of behaviour.

Similar assumptions are held about intelligence – 'born that way', 'runs in the family'. As Burr points out:

> This view of personality, then, suggests that the kind of person you are is in some degree the result of your biology (perhaps inherited through your genetic make-up, through the balance of chemicals operating in the brain, or through hormones and so on). (1995, p. 20)

This is, indeed, a view that we are likely to hear expressed in some way on a daily basis, part of the diet of popular psychology. It seems embedded in the language that we use. 'Road rage', for instance, has connotations of a physical/biological condition – a pathology – and raises in yet another guise the old nature/nurture debate.

This view of a biologically determined self is essentialist; that is, human beings have an essence or fixed nature that explains behaviour (Burr 1995). We shall return to 'essentialism' later.

Reflections

Think about your understanding of yourself in terms of biology. In what circumstances and to what extent might you explain your behaviour and how you are as a person on grounds of biology? You might include, for instance, jealousy, sex drive, alcohol dependency, proneness to panic, stress or vertigo (so OK I'm beginning my own list!). Think too about the adequacy of biology as an explanation. To what extent can we transcend or overcome our biology? And what are the problems with this view of self?

Whilst we are undeniably embodied beings, this type of explanation of being in the social world is limited and limiting – or reductionist. Thinking that clearly puts notions of self into a broader frame comes from anthropological and cultural studies. Is the individualistic concept of self common to all cultures and all historical eras? Comparison of different societies suggests that the Western idea of personality and individualistic notions of the essential, unique self is not universal. A contrast has been made between individual/independent and collectivist/interdependent understandings of self (Gough & McFadden 2001). Cousins (1989) compared self-descriptions of people from Japan and from the USA. He analyzed statements made in response to the question 'Who am I?' and found that far more American subjects used 'pure psychological attributes', such as 'I am honest' or 'I am sociable'. Japanese people were more likely to use social role statements, such as 'a father' or 'a student'. The merging of self and society can also be found in the grammatical forms of the Japanese language. Inherent within everyday language use are kinds of identity and social relationships. Harré & Gillett (1994) have analyzed English and Japanese languages in terms of the use of personal pronouns, words referring to self and others. English has very few pronouns – I, me, you, she, they, etc. The Japanese language has approximately 260 ways of referring to different social relations. In Japanese '. . . it is *utterly impossible* to form a sentence without *also* commenting on the relationship between oneself and one's interlocutor' (Kondo 1990, p. 31).

It seems, then, that ' . . . comparison with Japan clarifies the individualistic emphasis in many western cultures such as the USA (the focus on individual achievement, individual expression, individual authenticity, autonomy and independence)' (Wetherell & Maybin 1996, p. 233). It is interesting to note, at this point, that critiques of the essentialist Western view of self as independent and detached from relationships and society have also arisen from the collective resistance of oppressed groups (including disabled people, women, lesbians and gays) and the emergence of what has been called 'identity politics'.

Once the common-sense view of self is questioned, however, many alternatives emerge and I can only begin to indicate some general patterns in portraits of self. One widely used concept is that of 'role', with the idea that what we do is, at least to an extent, context-bound and dependent on the role that we are currently occupying or playing. It highlights the impact of social expectations and situations on the self. My thoughts, feelings and perhaps even, like the character Wemmick in *Great Expectations*, the shape of my mouth changes as I return home from work, changing from a work to a family-member role. Goffman's work has been highly influential in suggesting a theatrical or 'dramaturgical' view of social actors rehearsing and reproducing various scripts provided by society. He developed a flexible notion of self as social process, a project of impression management:

> When an individual plays a part he implicitly requests his observers to take seriously the impression that is fostered before them. (1959, p. 77)

The concept of role can be helpful in linking personal identity with social life and how we negotiate and act out, in our own ways, expectations placed on us. Goffman offers a conception of self that is continuously negotiated within a complex weft and warp of relationships. There are, however, criticisms of this idea. It has been suggested that this concept of self remains basically individualistic: actors on a public stage in the pursuit of their private goals (Hallis 1977).

A view of self that is embedded in relationships and culture has emerged through the concept of narrative. From this perspective, narrative is a bridge between individual experience and culture. McLeod explains:

> We are born into a world of stories. A culture is structured around myths, legends, family tales and other stories that have existed since long before we are born, and will continue long after we die. We construct a personal identity by aligning ourselves with some of these stories, by 'dwelling within' them. (McLeod 1998a, p. 153)

I think immediately of family stories told repeatedly by grandparents to my children. A favourite concerns the time when the baby bath was filled and positioned in front of the fire and while the dad's back was turned two of them climbed into the bath fully clothed. It is a story of shared family history,

Reflections

Think about any experiences you might have had of taking on a 'sick role'. When people are ill, they are not only affected by the illness itself, they can take on a role of being ill, needing help, needing a social space for illness, and fulfilling their own and others' expectations of being ill. They can acquire an identity as a sick person and take on a 'sick role'. Being ill is a 'way of being' and behaving and when people are ill they act in ways that confirm that they are ill. Jot down a few words about your experiences of being ill. In what ways did your life change? Did you think of yourself differently and did others act differently towards you? Did you get help and support and how did you respond to help and support (or the lack of it)?

of mischievousness and my embarrassment, at least in Granny's version of the story. Gergen uses a telling quotation from Hardy (1968):

> We dream in narrative, daydream in narrative, remember, anticipate, hope, despair, believe, doubt, plan, revise, criticize, construct, gossip, learn, hate and love by narrative. (1999, p. 70)

The notion of narrative is of a continuing account of ourselves and the series of occurrences in our lives, to ourselves and others. Anderson (1997) says we understand and give meaning and intelligibility to our experiences through narrative or storytelling and she quotes Madison:

> The self is the way we relate, account for, speak about our actions. . . . The self is the unity of an ongoing narrative, a narrative which lasts a thousand and one nights and more – until, as Proust might say, that night arrives which is followed by no dawn. (1988, pp. 161–162)

Selves, then, are constructed through language and maintained in narrative. A self is not a thing inside an individual, but a process or activity that occurs in the dynamic space of communication between people (Freedman & Combs 1996). In this understanding of human beings, there is a move from the inwardness of an individual self, to 'being in the world' and 'relating in the world' with other human beings. The focus of interest is moved from the inside of an individual to the outside of the human world. Writing of the link between identity and narrative life history, Widdershoven states:

> What then is narrative identity? It is the unity of a person's life as it is experienced and articulated in stories that express this experience. . . . the unity of a person's life is dependent on being a character in an enacted narrative. We live our lives according to a script, which secures that our actions are part of a meaningful totality. Our actions are organized in such a way that we can give account of them, justify them by telling an intelligible story about them. (1993, p. 7)

Accounts are co-created. They are not only a way of understanding ourselves, relationships and social worlds, they fashion selves, relationships and social worlds. Stories are told with others: 'We are heavily dependent upon the willingness of co-actors in the construction of our stories' (Burr 1995, p. 136). Experiences are intertwined, given shape and meaning through stories that both form and inform. Granny's stories of the baby bath incident were explicitly co-authored with the children, through their addition of omitted details and correction of errors in recounted tales.

This accounting of actions can also project existing stories into a presumed future. Plot development can hold different possibilities, of course, although grounded in existing stories: 'I'm overburdened with my work and suppose I always will be, unless I change jobs, but I can't see that happening in the foreseeable future . . . etc'. Stories, however, can also narrate into a preferred future, e.g. 'I'm overburdened by work at the moment but there is a new member of staff starting soon and the opportunity to renegotiate my

---

Reflections

The idea of critical incidents has been drawn on in developing reflective practice by Lillyman (2000). A critical incident can be:

- an ordinary experience
- an experience that did not go to plan
- an incident that went well
- an incident that reflects the values and beliefs held by the practitioner
- an incident that highlights the expertise of the practitioner
- an incident that allows the identification of learning.

Pick out a moment or experience in your professional career or training that changed you or bore personal significance. Write down or tell your story. Reflect on the images and feelings it provokes. How has this event, and all it means to you, shaped your subsequent experiences and life events?

---

workload . . . etc'. Stories, then, guide action, make sense of what has happened, is happening, and will happen and guide us to act in certain ways and not others (Somers 1994, pp. 613–614).

Turning specifically to professionals' narratives, Mattingly has investigated the complex interconnections between narrative and experience in clinical work through the 'therapeutic narratives' of occupational therapists. She states that therapists:

> . . . operate with multiple storylines, multiple possible plots which point towards different possible selves, and they experiment with a variety of self understandings through the actions they take and the experiences they try to create for themselves and others. . . . (1998 p. 119)

Professionals construct narratives as stories of themselves, their roles, and their practice. Professionals are particularly likely to tell stories to make sense of difficult relationships, interrelations and points of conflict with others, managers, colleagues and clients. Mattingly emphasizes the dramas that underlie encounters in therapy when there are collisions between expectations and intentions, and unfolding events with others, particularly when desires run high creating significant experiences.

Self, then, is 'itself' constructed within the wider social and historical context and in the local context of our daily lives as we move between and within (in my case) being a father, husband, lecturer, friend, researcher, man, white, middle-aged, disabled and the list continues. This 'self-pluralistic approach' denies the subjective 'reality' of my self:

> Rather, it postulates an individual who encounters his or her world from a plurality of positions, through a plurality of voices, in relation to a plurality of self-concepts, yet who still retains a meaningful coherence. . . . (Cooper & Rowan 1999, p. 2)

Reflections

There is much that we can draw on in building and maintaining a sense of self including: our religious beliefs, our nationalities, our political allegiances, our sexual preferences, the clothes we wear, our hairstyles, the food we eat, the music we listen to and our possessions. There is much too that can undermine our sense of self or personal resources in communicating and sustaining identity: the onset of illness, the loss of employment, changing partners, the loss of family members and, speaking personally, children moving into adulthood and moving away from home. Think of yourself – discuss with a partner – and make a few written notes on the following:

- Why is a sense of identity important to you?
- What factors do you draw on in your sense of self?
- What factors and circumstances threaten your sense of self?
- How do you communicate your sense of identity to strangers, in close relationships, in professional relationships?

Identity is an active project for each person but contained and defined within available resources and choices.

YOU AND I: UNDERSTANDING COMMUNICATION

We have looked at ways of understanding 'I' that cannot be divorced from understandings of 'you and I'. From this point of view, concepts of self cannot be addressed separately from concepts of communication and relationships. Not surprisingly, then, the notion of personal relationships can be seen as irrevocably intertwined with communication. Communication is a means of expressing a relationship; it constitutes the initiation, maintenance and ending of a relationship, and it is the medium and substance through which the relationship is defined and given meaning (VanderVoort & Duck 2000). This is not, of course, confined to verbal communication. It encompasses what we do to and for each other. A kiss or slap can certainly change a relationship. Communication is central to our personal lives, and also to our collective or social lives, being the medium through which societies work.

Given the complexity of communication, it is hardly surprising that there are numerous definitions and ways of understanding the processes, almost as many as there are people who provide definitions. However, there seems to be a dominant way of looking at communication that seems to accord with common sense – that is, as a process of sending and receiving messages. Rungapadiachy adopts such a model suggesting that most social and behavioural theorists would agree on the same basic model. In its entirety, the most popular communication model that is used is as follows:

1. Sender (self)
2. Encoder (converting thought into message)
3. Channel (verbal, non-verbal, both verbal and non-verbal)
4. Decoder (interpretation of message)
5. Receiver (other/others). (1999, p. 195)

Some definitions concentrate more on the communication process itself, rather than the notion of message sending. Hartley, for instance, bases his approach on Clampitt's model of communication as dance:

> This uses the analogy of a dance where partners have to coordinate their movements and arrive at a mutual understanding of where they are going. There are rules and skills but there are also flexibilities – dancers can inject their own style into the movements. (Hartley 1999, p. 18)

Hartley broadens the basic model in terms of different contexts: the nature of the audience, relationship between the participants, and medium or channel of communication. As to the last of these, in more recent years the rapid uptake of mobile phones has been something of a revolution in channels of communication, and not just verbally; texting has even led to the development of something of a new language of symbols.

Many skills-based approaches are based on a 'sending and receiving messages' model and involve identifying small discernible elements or units of interpersonal communication, such as eye contact or use of questions, which can then be analyzed in terms of the effectiveness of communication and incorporated into training packages.

The 'sending and receiving messages' view of communication seems to me to be a common-sense view, with perhaps particular relevance to present-day Western societies. We are, for instance, bombarded by adverts for products – designer label clothing, scents and deodorants, cars, drinks, food – on the grounds of the messages we can convey about ourselves – be cool, be sexy, be male.

Nevertheless, this view of communication has been challenged from a number of viewpoints that might be encompassed within the umbrella of

Reflections

Think of communication in terms of sending messages. In an interaction with another person how do you send messages, and what about you sends messages (both deliberately and unintentionally)? Make a list of all the channels of communication. Your list should include non-verbal behaviours, body language, appearance, etc. Having used this activity with students, I have found that the category most often omitted is the quality of speech (pitch, stress – you might add others in your list).

'dynamic' or 'shared meaning' models. There are a number of important aspects to a dynamic model of communication. It is a rejection of models of communication conceived as the sending and receiving, or transmission, of information. From the viewpoint of a dynamic model, communication is seen as a trans–action constructed between people. It is an interplay between people in which participants are both active agents, effecting the interplay, and re-active agents, effected by the interplay. There is no simple one-to-one correspondence between acts of communication and the meaning expressed. The context is all important, giving and given meaning. Even signals that might seem to have a well-defined meaning, such as raising the hand to signal 'stop', depend on the context of the two-way flow. If accompanied by a smile, for instance, the raising of the hand could be meant as and understood to be a joke. Furthermore, there are differences between cultures in the actual behaviours used and their possible meanings. Robinson states that:

> Despite policy initiatives, there is abundant evidence that the health service and health practitioners do not always meet the communication needs of minority ethnic patients effectively. (2002, p. 1)

In understanding the diversity of communication needs, a more holistic view looks beyond the messages sent and received in 'atomistic units'–that is, specific behaviours. Pearce writes:

Reflections

Consider the following statement: 'Please do these exercises at least twice a day, though stop if it gets too painful'. (You may have assumed that the statement is made by the physiotherapist to the client.) In this example, the intention is to establish the treatment regime as planned by the physiotherapist. This statement can certainly be thought of in terms of sending a message. However, think about it in terms of its meaning in the context of the professional–client relationship. What are the different possibilities?

The action, in terms of the professional–client relationship, will obviously depend on the existing relationship between the physiotherapist and the client, and their history of communication, i.e. whether the relationship is being defined, maintained or redefined. The crucial point is that the relationship dimension provides the context for the meaning of the content dimension. The client can interpret the content in many ways. If, for instance, there is a trusting relationship, the client may interpret this as a useful suggestion to which he or she should comply. If, on the other hand, their relationship is distant, and the client feels the physiotherapist has no real knowledge of him or her as a person, this might be seen as a rigid directive more to do with the physiotherapist complying with the expectations of the professional role. The meaning too will depend on the client's history of experiences with professionals.

This social constructionist perspective on conversation requires us to think in terms of interactive patterns, not atomistic units. . . . we must treat conversations – and clusters of conversations – as systems in which the whole is different from the sum of the parts. (1994, pp. 23–25)

Within this perspective, 'discourse always has an *action orientation*' (Wetherell & Maybin 1996, p. 244). Speech, writing and non-verbal communication are forms of social action. Social relationships are achieved through and enmeshed within interpersonal communication. Relationships between physiotherapist and client are defined or maintained through the communication between them.

WE: UNDERSTANDING SOCIAL RELATIONS

'We' implicitly connotes 'other'/'not-we'. Group identity is 'in relation to'. To be a professional has meaning in relation to non-professionals or lay people. We live in a society of social divisions within which 'we' define and are defined: male/female, disabled/non-disabled, young/old, working/-middle/upper class, gay/straight. Inherent within this understanding of society is some notion of power. I spent my youth in Beeston, Leeds, and knew well the graveyard that is the setting for Tony Harrison's poem *V*, and these verses are, for me, an affective starting point for considering social relations. His Vs are contested power relations, much more effectively expressed in poetry than in the jargon of the social sciences.

These Vs are the versuses of life
from LEEDS v. DERBY, Black/White
and (as I've known to my cost) man v. wife,
Communist v. Fascist, Left v. Right,

Class v. class as bitter as before,
the unending violence of US and THEM,
personified in 1984
by Coal Board MacGregor and the NUM,

Hindu/Sikh, body/soul, heart v. mind,
East/West, male/female, and the ground
these fixtures are fought out on 's Man, resigned
to hope from his future what his past never found. (1987)

Payne (2000, p. 1) claims that the idea of social divisions is one of the most useful and powerful tools available in understanding ourselves, society and why society operates as it does. Payne (2000, pp. 242–243) social divisions as being society-wide distinctions between two or more groups of people that, among other things:

- are perceived as being substantially different materially or culturally
- are long-standing and sustained by dominant cultural beliefs, the organization of social institutions and individual interaction

- confer unequal access to resources – and thus different life chances and styles
- engender shared identities in terms of perceived difference from those in an alternative category of the same social division.

Identity and social division are closely interconnected issues and have increasingly come to prominence in areas of inquiry across the social sciences (Hetherington 1998). Our sense of who we are, our own identity in relation to (sometimes 'versus') the identity of others, is part and parcel of our lived experience and interwoven, and created within, our interactions with others. Our sense of who we are is linked, for instance, to our awareness of our identities as women or as men. Both gender and sexuality can play a significant role in our understanding of identity, but, of course, what it means to be a man or woman, heterosexual or homosexual, also depends on the society we live in. Identity is at the interface between the personal (thoughts, feelings, personal histories) and the social (the societies in which we live and the social, cultural and economic factors that shape experience and make it possible for people to take up some identities and render others inaccessible or impossible) (Woodward 2000, p. 18).

Questions of identity, then, take analysis into the political arena. Jenkins writes of resistance as potent affirmation of group identity:

> Struggles for a different allocation of resources and resistance to categorisation are one and the same thing. . . . Whether or not there is an explicit call to arms in these terms, something that can be called self-assertion – or 'human spirit' is at the core of resistance to domination . . . It is as intrinsic, and as necessary, to that social life as the socialising tyranny of categorisation. (1996, p. 175)

Similarly, Hetherington suggests that identity has become significant through resistance to dominance in unequal power relations:

> One of the main issues behind this interest in identity and in identity politics more generally has been the relationship between marginalisation and a politics of resistance, and affirmative, empowering choices of identity and a politics of difference. (1998, p. 21)

Politics of difference can divide society into opposing groups, into 'them and us' and 'self and other', and where there is difference there is the potential for institutionalized discrimination (Thompson 2001) – that is, the unfair or unequal treatment of individuals or groups that is built into institutional organizations, policies, and practices at personal, environmental and structural levels (Swain et al. 1998). It is a process through which groups and individuals experience different forms of oppression, including racism, sexism, ageism, disablism and so on. To take sexism as an example, Abbott (2000) demonstrates a whole range of gender inequalities in employment and pensions, state benefits, labour market access and the poverty experienced by lone–parent families. Work plays a key role. Despite other changes in paid employment patterns, women's earnings are still substantially lower than men's

(Hatt 2000). Domestic work, including unpaid caring work, remains devalued and predominantly 'women's work'. Thompson (2001, p. 140) suggests that forms of oppression can impact on identity in a number of ways:

1. alienation, isolation and marginalization – social exclusion from full participation in society
2. economic position and life chances
3. confidence, self-esteem and aspirations
4. social aspirations, career opportunities and so on.

Concern about identity is also concern about change: challenging social expectations about identity, establishing new identities and transforming existing identities (Jenkins 1996). Since the 1950s 'new social movements', including the women's movement, the black power movement and the disabled people's movement, have played a significant role in the politics of identity. They can be seen as collective endeavours to give voice to and affirm new identities. It is apparent that the more overt the discrimination and oppression that people experience, the more heightened their awareness and sense of vulnerability around that particular identity. Monks states:

> People who are socially excluded and oppressed, and who are often also defined as lacking qualities of a normative social being, may find solidarity in the shared experience of exclusion itself. . . . The 'communities' which emerge may become politically active . . . Experience of the interdependence, mutuality and solidarity which arise from shared activities and communication is an important part of membership, even of direct political action. (1999, p 71)

I am writing this on 11th September 2002, the anniversary of what is, for many, a momentous event in defining identity collectively and individually – us versus them. The extract from Harrison's poem, above, begins with the line: 'These Vs are the versuses of life'. As the events of 11th September 2001 and the continuing aftermath illustrate, these are the versuses of death as well as life.

For many social scientists the broad picture is one of fractured, fluid, multiple and contested identities. According to Bradley (1996, p. 23), for instance, people can draw their sense of identity from a broad range of sources, including class, gender, age, marital status, sexual preference, consumption patterns and disability. Furthermore, identity is a matter of 'becoming' rather than simply 'being':

> Far from being eternally fixed in some essentialized past, they are subject to the continuous 'play' of history, culture and power. . . . identities are the names we give to the different ways we are positioned by, and position ourselves within, the narratives of the past. (Hall 1990, p. 225)

Reflections

Can you think of any problems there might be in 'dualistic thinking' (in terms of binary oppositions such as black/white, woman/man and so on)?

As Braham & Janes (2001) suggest, recognition of the complexity of differences within and between divisions points towards the celebration of difference and away from concentration on collective, structural disadvantage and inequality. Within divisions, for instance, the 'butch' lesbian, the drag queen, transvestite and 'macho' gay problematize sex and gender categories (Butler 1989). There are multiple gender identities, masculinities and femininities, rather than one masculine and one feminine type. In any society there is a whole range of ways in which femininity and masculinity can be expressed. Differences between divisions become problematic through the recognition that we are all a complex amalgam of multiple aspects of identity and members of several different socially divided groups. Social divisions are not simply additive either in terms of disadvantage or identity. Black disabled women, for instance, experience discriminations that can connect, overlap and reinforce each other – by being black and disabled and female. Membership of different socially divided groups can also operate in contradictory and complex ways (Vernon & Swain 2002).

In a context of diversity and fluidity, identity is contested within conflicts of interest and power inequalities. Williams shows how the commonality between women stressed by feminism in the 1970s has been challenged:

> Feminism based on black, lesbian and disabled politics has pointed to the need to deconstruct the category of 'woman' in order to understand the complex and inter-connected range of identities and subject positions through which women's experiences are constituted, as well as the ways these also change over time and place. (1996, p. 69)

This is a feature of most social movements. It is, perhaps, ironic that the very context in which people can become united is also a context in which divisions are affirmed. Thus, Lorde has stated:

> Somewhere on the edge of consciousness, there is what I call a *mythical norm* ... this norm is usually defined as white, thin, male, young, heterosexual, Christian and financially secure. It is with this mythical norm that the trappings of power reside within this society. Those of us who stand outside that power often identify one way in which we are different, and we assume that to be the primary cause of all oppression, forgetting other distortions around difference, some of which we ourselves may be practising. (1984, p. 37)

From this viewpoint, oppression becomes much more diffuse than the idea that there are people who are oppressed and there are others who oppress. It is possible to be both oppressed and oppressor.

Reflections

1. Thinking of yourself, what would you say are the main determinants of your identity, however you would define it?
2. How have identities changed in Western societies over the past, say, 50 years? Think particularly of gender identities, what it meant to be a man or a woman in Britain just after the Second World War and what it means now.
3. Do you recognize yourself as both oppressed and oppressor? With whom and why?

Chapter 2

The professional context

Frances Reynolds

There is increasing evidence that effective health care depends not only on the technical expertise of health professionals, but also on the quality of the communications that occur in every aspect of the health-care context, and the nature of the relationships that are to be found there. This chapter explores the notions of empowering and enabling relationships. It examines some of the opportunities and barriers to effective partnership with clients, that arise not so much from the individual skills (or lack of skills) of therapists, but from the traditional conceptual lenses through which illness and disability are viewed, and from certain forces within the heath- and social-care systems. Enabling and therapeutic communications with clients are jeopardized by the prevalence of disabling models of care, unexamined assumptions about normality, long-standing organizational barriers to partnership approaches with clients, and pervasive notions of health and treatment that focus on pathology rather than quality of life. The attitudes, skills and motivation of individual therapists are not the only factors that determine whether effective, enabling communications occur or not.

The professional contexts in which therapists work contain forces that tend to inhibit truly enabling communications with clients. Personal factors such as stereotyped attitudes also limit therapists' ability to create genuine partnerships with their clients. Whilst many individual therapists value empowering relationships, they encounter significant barriers because of the ways in which health, disability, normality and well-being are defined in the health-care system, and in Western culture more generally. Effective and enabling communications depend as much on therapists having a critical awareness of these barriers as on their practice of skilful non-verbal and verbal strategies of interaction. In addition, therapists need to recognize that clients/users of health services have a wide range of needs and goals, and do not always have agendas that coincide with those of health professionals. The key argument within this chapter is that professional, organizational and societal contexts create considerable difficulties for clients themselves, as well as for the health professionals who are endeavouring to work in non-discriminatory and empowering ways. Through awareness of these difficulties, therapists can take steps to enhance their working partnerships with clients.

Therapists' ways of working with people who have long-term impairments or illness (rather than acute conditions) are the focus of this chapter. Enabling communications are particularly vital – and frequently problematic – for those who come into contact with health professionals over long periods of time. Their needs for enabling communications are pressing yet often unmet.

ENABLING RELATIONSHIPS

Empowerment would seem at first sight to involve some transmission of power from health professional to client. Health professionals sometimes express reluctance to give clients real power in the rehabilitation process for a number of reasons. For example, they may doubt that clients have the necessary expertise to make informed decisions, they may wish to preserve their own professional status and they may feel threatened by any perceived short-coming or criticism by users of services (as reviewed by Hickey & Kipping 1998). Many health professionals themselves work in disempowering circumstances and, therefore, find it difficult to empower their clients (Trnobranski 1994). Some fear that user involvement will further increase their heavy workloads (Poulton 1999). They may also wish to avoid allowing clients to do themselves harm (for example, by refusing an effective but painful treatment) because of their professional code of practice. Given that clients are individuals with different needs, resources, and vulnerabilities, an approach to empowerment that has received much attention is the *partnership* approach to therapy.

Enabling relationships as partnerships

A *partnership* approach to health care and rehabilitation makes certain assumptions. Both the professional and the client are regarded as bringing strengths or resources to the therapeutic process, and the therapeutic relationship. At times, the therapist may provide more of certain resources (such as expert knowledge), but at other points in the therapy process the client offers the more significant resources for advancing change, e.g. social support, skills, or the aspirations that motivate engagement in rehabilitation. The professional and the client together are part of the team that will openly share information and make decisions about the way forwards in therapy/rehabilitation. The relationship is respectful and affirmative, rather than shaped by dependency, submissiveness or power struggles (Thompson 2001); it is also based on adult strategies of communication, rather than infantalizing, manipulation or stereotyping, with both partners having a respected voice in the interaction. The client is, therefore, motivated to share responsibility with the therapist for the therapy process and outcome. The purpose of the partnership is to promote the client's self-actualization, development and quality of life, rather than pressurizing specifically for better compliance with treatment.

Whilst many disabled people welcome partnership approaches (Edwards 2002), it is important to respect individual differences in clients' preferences and assumptions. Particularly in the early stages of illness or following trauma, some clients feel too shocked or too unwell to make decisions or to take responsibility within the therapy process. Feelings of depression, hopelessness or fear may dominate. Some may feel ill-equipped to offer an informed opinion (Biley 1992). Some individuals for whom hospitalization or therapy is a new and perhaps threatening experience, may lack the confidence to ask questions or seek information (Cegala et al. 2000). Many disabled people, however, with extensive experience of living with their impairment are very well informed and clear about their needs and goals. Other individuals experience both good days and bad days, needing therapists to provide support and treatment at some points, for example during an exacerbation of their illness, but to provide more of a consultancy role at other points (Charmaz 1991, Duggan & Dijkers 1999). It is important for therapists to avoid making decisions 'for' a disabled person who is in a state of vulnerability, as such decisions can have undesirable long-term consequences. A therapist adopting a partnership approach needs to be sensitive to the client's expressed feelings and preferences, ensuring that the client can take on control and responsibility as and when ready to do so. To do this skilfully, however, the therapist requires a high level of reflective understanding of the barriers to partnership – conceptual, organizational and personal.

CONCEPTUAL BARRIERS TO PARTNERSHIP: THE BIOMEDICAL MODEL OF HEALTH AND HEALTH CARE

A substantial barrier to communication within the health-care and therapy context is the traditional biomedical view of illness and disability. This conceptual model presents the body in terms of a complex machine requiring attention when parts and processes function 'abnormally'. Whilst this viewpoint has undoubtedly led to a huge growth in biological knowledge and an awesome capacity to intervene medically in certain biological processes, it has distracted attention away from the importance of the communication processes occurring between professionals and clients. The biomedical conceptualization of disease and impairment has traditionally encouraged clinicians to listen to clients only in so far as they can shed clues on their pathology and thereby contribute to an effective diagnosis. Even in mental-health settings, where disease and pathology are less obviously relevant, the biomedical model still has a dominant influence over diagnosis and treatment.

An unfortunate consequence of the biomedical model has been the neglect, until recently, of communication skills training among doctors and therapists. If disease, disability and diagnosis are framed squarely in terms of body pathology, then individual experience, values and goals seem quite irrelevant to decisions about treatment, care and support. Also clients' roles in decision-making about treatment become marginalized within this perspective, as they are not considered to have the requisite biomedical knowledge to offer informed opinions. Furthermore, the biomedical model has been associated with power relationships and social status within the health-care context. It appears that those regarded as having the greatest power to 'cure' disease (i.e. medical practitioners) are accorded the greatest status. Professionals who contribute to care, support or rehabilitation have been seen, at least until recently, as having a lower status 'supplementary' to medicine. In the lowest position within the hierarchy of power have been clients, as their role within this conceptual framework is simply to present diseased or injured bodies for medical attention. Their subjective voice, their experience of living with illness or impairment, their resourcefulness and their very status as persons of worth have all too often been disregarded, particularly within the publicly funded health system. Only recently have medical and other health-care students been encouraged to really listen to clients' own accounts of their illness experiences in order to develop empathy and insight. Kirklin (2001, p. 11) reported that one of her students described the marked difference in the experience of fully listening to a client and taking a medical history: 'Taking a history is black and white. Listening to the patient's story adds the colour'.

A further oppressive force associated with the biomedical perspective has been the restrictive definition of 'normality', which in turn drives many of the goals of therapy. Until the challenge in recent years presented by the disabled people's movement, clients with impairments have been thought simply to aspire to a return to full physical functioning and physical independence. Whilst it is important to acknowledge that some affected people retain these aspirations, others challenge the view that satisfaction with one's life and body need be directly related to one's degree of physical functioning. Instead, they re-prioritize their activities and goals (Weitzenkamp et al. 2000), and over time reconstruct different, yet equally positive, identities (Swain & French 2000). When working with disabled people, it is clearly necessary to listen without prejudgement to the person's own views and aspirations. Whereas one person might be motivated to return to the former roles and responsibilities that he/she associates with a 'normal' life, another might regard quality of life as dependent on forging alternative meaningful strategies of living. I recently interviewed a number of women about their strategies of achieving a satisfactory quality of life with multiple sclerosis (MS). One interviewee described a strategy that clearly did not involve carrying out a large number of the tasks involved in 'independent' living. Perhaps as a result of such altered priorities, she judged her quality of life to be very good:

> You find functional strategies, pay people to do the things that are boring, that you don't want to waste your energy on, so now I pay somebody to do my cleaning, I pay somebody to do the ironing, I pay somebody to do the heavy gardening. Quite a lot of that goes on paying people to do things, but if I've got limited energy I'm not going to waste it on ironing shirts (pause) and I think if one were in the business of giving out advice, which one mustn't do, but should you be, that would be

the piece of advice that I'd give anybody, do not waste your very limited energy on things that are boring.

Prevalent conceptual perspectives on the ill and disabled body that emphasize loss of normality and moral worth are clearly profoundly disempowering. For clients with acute conditions, medical and therapeutic treatments often prove effective within a short period of time. Their negative social positioning in the client role may be tiresome or even infuriating, but at least it is short lived. However, for people with chronic conditions or life-long differences in bodily functioning, the regular encounter with disempowering and sometimes profoundly unethical professional assumptions and practices may be a significant source of distress. Atkinson argues:

> As 'deficit' theories (the measurement of differences) came into vogue first in medicine and psychology, but later in education, people were seen as cases to be treated or specially trained. The voices of people themselves were replaced by their case histories, prepared by others on their behalf. . . . (1999, p. 13).

Given the history of disempowerment within the medical and social-care system, it is clear that the recent initiatives to involve clients in partnerships and to promote collaborative, enabling communications are huge and radical challenges.

THE ORGANIZATIONAL CONTEXT

There are certain factors within the current National Health Service (NHS) that are encouraging partnership approaches to working with clients. The NHS is currently advocating an empowerment or partnership model of helping relationships in which the client's (and carer's) voice is heard, and where health professionals and clients work collaboratively with agreed, shared agendas (see Holman & Lorig 2000 for one discussion). User involvement in service planning and evaluation is also being encouraged (see current NHS website http://www.nhs.uk/patientsvoice/core-principles. asp). The wider consumer culture, and the social forces created by the disabled people's movement, have encouraged this partnership approach. Evidence suggests that when clients are genuinely included in the decision-making process, with their views, experiences and goals acknowledged, and their questions answered, then they are more committed to engaging in therapy, and are more satisfied with the therapeutic process and outcome (Ley 1988).

Whilst the partnership approach to care represents an admirable goal, it is one that is not easy to achieve. If health professionals are to communicate in a genuinely enabling or therapeutic manner, they do not just require a high level of interpersonal skill and sensitivity. In addition, they need to be aware of the disabling barriers presented within the wider organizational and cultural context, because these readily and profoundly influence therapists' interpersonal encounters with clients.

Reflections

Either from your experience in the clinical placement setting, or from your general observations as a client, draw up some of the organizational barriers that seem to exist in the NHS, which make it difficult for therapists (and other staff) to establish genuine partnerships between clients. Ignore the personal motivation of doctors and therapists and instead consider factors within the organization of health care that impede partnership approaches. If possible, compare your views and experiences with those identified by a colleague.

Numerous organizational barriers to enabling communications within health care exist. You may have identified several. For example:

- The lengthy professional training and socialization of health workers sets up 'social distance' from clients.
- Social constructions of health and health care tend to encourage a focus on pathology, and treatment, rather than considering clients as individuals (for example, a client may be regarded as a 'head injury' rather than a person with a unique biography, roles, relationships, and so on).
- Resource limitations result in brief appointments, waiting lists, rationing and withdrawal of certain services, regardless of clients' needs and preferences.
- Some of the values and assumptions driving evidence-based health-care practice risk distracting attention away from the quality of health-care relationships.

Without awareness of these and other organizational barriers, relationships are likely to be incongruent, and both client and professional may experience frustration, or disillusionment as a result. These factors will receive further discussion below.

A substantial barrier to the creation of genuinely collaborative relationships with clients is created by the very lengthy professional socialization of all health professionals. This undoubtedly delivers a high level of skill and knowledge that necessarily has to underpin a variety of effective interventions. As an unwanted side effect, however, this lengthy socialization, together with their 'caring' responsibilities, may inculcate health professionals with negative views of disability and a limited understanding of clients' personal resources for managing their lives. For example, French (1994) has shown that health professionals' attitudes towards disabled people are no more 'enlightened' than those expressed by the lay population. Some disabled people who work in health care have commented on the negativity which they have directly experienced, albeit sometimes clothed in sympathetic concern (Iezzoni 1998). Basnett, a medical doctor who suffered a spinal injury later in his career, offers a sober reflection on his changing view of disability, once personally affected. He argues that the lengthy training of health professionals, together with their experience of working with people only when they are in need of treatment (and not when they are well or coping) means that ' . . . health professionals can develop a view of disability that is at substantial variance from its reality for many disabled people' (2001, p. 451).

The organizational context, particularly within the NHS, is highly complex because it relies on the co-ordination of effort among many different professional groups, each with rather different priorities, conceptual frameworks and modes of practice. For example, occupational therapists are more explicitly client-centred in their practice than physiotherapists (Sumsion et al. 1999). It is also a markedly resource-limited environment, so it is not surprising that professional groups sometimes perceive competition with each other for the resources to do their jobs effectively. The NHS is advocating a partnership approach, not only between health professionals and clients, but also among professionals of different disciplines. The goal is to provide a seamless service in which multi-disciplinary teams work together to provide maximally effective interventions for clients. Despite these laudable aims, professionals themselves often find it difficult to work co-operatively with colleagues from other disciplines (Miller et al. 2001). Their distinctive professional allegiances, developed over at least 3 years of training, cut across institutional boundaries (Øvretveit et al. 1997). When the roles of other professions are poorly understood, rivalry and miscommunication become extremely likely.

The organizational context can also impede enabling relationships through setting up health professionals as 'gatekeepers', rationing limited resources to clients. Inadequate budgets, for instance, may force occupational therapists to limit the provision of aids and adaptations that they know would make a great deal of difference to a client's quality of life. Even if therapists have the personal skills to work in an enabling way with clients to identify their needs and priorities, the physical and economic resources that should underpin health and social care may not be available. Therapists and clients are likely to experience much frustration if the required interventions, such as equipment, adaptations, additional physiotherapy or counselling support, are not accessible, particularly when they are recognized to help maximize quality of life. They can even save NHS resources in the longer term.

In the NHS, the boundaries of the organizational context are not to be located at the doors of hospitals and clinics. Because it is a publicly financed organization, there are economic and governmental pressures on health professionals that limit empowering practice. Government targets and deadlines (e.g. to reduce waiting lists) inevitably impact not only on the wider organization, but also on individual encounters between a therapist and a client. For example, pressures on appointment times may encourage therapists to focus narrowly on biomedical or functional issues, and to ignore the wider psychosocial problems that the client is experiencing.

Reflections

Read the following example of poor communication and consider organizational factors (rather than individual skill deficits) that might have acted as a barrier to communication:

> Margaret was examined by her consultant neurologist. She had been diagnosed with multiple sclerosis 4 years previously and was currently having increasing difficulty with her balance, mobility, and continence. At the end of the consultation, as the neurologist was preparing to leave, Margaret asked 'Could you suggest anything to help my balance?' The neurologist said rather abruptly as he exited from the room 'Try using a stick'. He shut the door behind him. The stick that she already used to assist her balance was under the plinth. The neurologist had not noticed this.

This interaction was clearly not enabling. The neurologist even appears to be overtly disrespectful. Whilst it is possible that the consultant neurologist had failed to acquire certain rudimentary communication skills, it is also possible that the organizational context inhibited a receptive attitude and genuine engagement with the client's question.

First, consider the pressures of time. Consultations between clients and medical and therapy staff are often required to be restricted to 6 minutes or so, which reduces the possibility of building rapport, and negotiating a shared agenda, as well as limiting opportunities for sensitive observation. The professional socialization that the consultant has received may have led to dismissive attitudes towards clients' concerns, hopes and levels of expertise about their illness. He might believe that his client was still hoping for a medical 'cure' for an untreatable illness, and that her question reflected this forlorn hope. Resource limitations may make health professionals feel defensive about unmet needs and, therefore, impatient with those who seem to be requesting additional support or treatment. These organizational pressures are not 'excuses' for rude or patronizing interactions with clients, but they suggest that enabling communications require reflective evaluation of the barriers set in place by the wider context. Otherwise, even the most individually skilled communicators will inevitably feel inhibited and frustrated by the constraints that they experience regularly in their encounters with clients.

There are also organizational pressures, possibly driven by the unexamined assumptions of the biomedical model, to value physical recovery over enhanced empowerment or quality of life when working with clients who have physical illness or impairment. This may be defensible in the case of short-lived, treatable physical conditions, but militates against taking the more holistic approach that people living with chronic conditions find helpful. Indeed, therapists who give priority to hearing their clients' concerns as a central facilitator of the rehabilitation process may even experience censure

Reflections

In reading the interaction between Margaret and her neurologist above, suggest some enabling communications that might have occurred, even in a brief encounter lasting only a minute or two. Consider some of the questions, information, and non-verbal communications that would have been more respectful and helpful to the client. If possible, discuss your ideas with others.

from colleagues for wasting time. A therapist who feels that he or she is paid to 'do physiotherapy', for example, may find it difficult to defend spending much of a treatment session listening to a client's concerns, even though this may prove to be beneficial in the longer term (Reynolds 1999a). Yet further training in counselling skills may result in therapists' increased confidence that listening to their clients is a productive and justifiable use of time.

There has been a tendency for many years to label people as 'different', who have physical impairment, behavioural disturbance or learning difficulties. Even in many cases where the person was healthy, and perhaps quite satisfied with their living arrangements, such difference ensured that a high degree of medical control could be exerted over his or her life. Many disabled people have experience of medical examinations that govern their schooling, financial supports and other entitlements. Such arrangements foster a societal view of disabled people and people who are chronically ill as 'other', dependent, tragic, or even less than human. The unexamined categorization of the client as other, and fundamentally different from health professionals, is further encouraged by the lack of representation of disabled people in the health professions. With the organizational context dominated by people who are highly educated, and non-disabled, a considerable social distance between professionals and clients is created. Such social distance may be another promoter of disabling attitudes, as it is only when people have opportunities to mix on an equal footing with others that stereotypes start to break down (Basnett 2001). The typical use of the term 'patient' seems to place the person so labelled as an 'object', masking individuals' vulnerabilities, strengths, goals and strategies for adapting to impairment or illness, and reducing the possibility that the therapist will make a genuine human connection with the users of their services. Applying unexamined terms such as 'multiple sclerosis victim' to a person, or describing an individual as 'confined' to a wheelchair also demean and disparage the users of services (Morris 1991). Patients all too often feel stripped of their individuality and skills when in hospital settings (Nichols 1989) and are intimidated by the knowledge and status that they ascribe to health professionals.

New initiatives in the professional context such as evidence-based practice (EBP) have laudable aims, in that it is clearly wasteful of everyone's efforts to be involved in treatments that lack any effectiveness (Reynolds & Trinder 2000). Even so, it is interesting that EBP, despite its wider social, economic and professional support, may have unintended consequences. EBP threatens to 'uniformize' treatments, based on scientific (usually quantitative) evidence about average treatment outcomes for groups of clients, and limiting client choice (Rogers 2002). Yet the verbal and non-verbal interactions between health professional and individual client are rarely subject to scientific evaluation. Because EBP, by definition, is usually grounded in group outcomes, there is the risk that the individual client's agendas, needs and resources will be overlooked during encounters with therapists, threatening genuine partnership.

So what are the implications of the organizational context for communication and enabling relationships? Clearly there are a number of barriers to respectful and open communication despite the recent rhetoric advocating 'partnership'. The organizational context, including its history over the last century, does not in reality do much to encourage clients and professionals to meet as human beings. Instead, they are placed in complementary roles as representatives of dominant social groups, each with a tendency to see the partner in the relationship as other, and socially different. Health-care workers have traditionally been professionally socialized to view the lack of objectivity and scientific knowledge of the client as problematic, because these are the qualities valued in so much of their training. Lengthy training also makes communication more difficult as technical terms and medical jargon that come to be well understood by therapists often create confusion for clients. Governmental and institutional pressures to treat clients with utmost efficiency also militate against open and enabling interactions. Clients, too, have often been socialized into perceiving health professionals as extremely busy and as occupying a high status, powerful position. Such perceptions can work to inhibit their disclosures, and to encourage passivity. The effects of illness, trauma and emotional turmoil can also inhibit the clients' communications, and ability to work in partnership.

CONCLUSIONS

This chapter has encouraged you to consider a wide range of barriers to creating enabling relationships with clients. The conceptual rigidity of the biomedical model of health and health care has traditionally rendered clients as passive, to be assessed and treated by health professionals, with little influence over the processes involved. Whilst many health-care systems, including the NHS, are now advocating partnership approaches, a number of organizational barriers continue to exist. Factors such as traditional professional and client roles, the social distance between therapist and client, time and resource limitations all conspire to limit genuine partnership and open communication. To overcome the various conceptual and organizational barriers to genuine partnership, individual therapists might consider a variety of strategies. They may try engaging in critical reflection, which will include reflective examination of the clinical environment, organizational policies and other relevant factors shaping local health care and therapy practice.

Challenging the operation of the biomedical model of health, illness and disability in the local context is a good strategy, and educating team members (including doctors) about the more empowering psychosocial and social models. It is important to listen to clients and work proactively to include their views in service planning and service evaluation. It also helps to read literature, whether qualitative research or autobiography, that provides insider views of the experience of illness and disability, including reflective analyses of the impact that such stories make on oneself (Kirklin 2001). Such insights may increase empathy and challenge negative stereotypes of disability, including the tragic and victim conceptualizations that many disabled people reject. Encouraging seminars and other forms of discussion within the whole team is a good way to highlight disabling assumptions and discriminatory practices within the services provided. It is also important to work proactively to increase support and cohesiveness within the clinical team, as support reduces burnout and helps team members to remain emotionally available to clients. It is useful to set up and use regular clinical supervision sessions, or co-counselling sessions with peers, during which any emotional and other difficulties arising from work with clients can be worked through without incurring judgements about 'not coping'.

Many books on counselling and communication skills focus exclusively on individual attitudes and interactive behaviours. Your relationships with clients will certainly benefit from an enhanced repertoire of skills for listening and responding to clients. Some clients benefit considerably if you have additional skills for appropriately motivating and educating them. Other chapters in this book aim to assist you in increasing your skills repertoire. However, it is also important to consider the wider cultural and organizational context, because forces beyond the individual therapist and client influence the patterns of relationship that they establish. To foster enabling relationships with clients, the therapist will need to harness personal skills *and* organizational supports, whilst also challenging the diverse forces operating in the wider environment that inhibit therapist–client partnerships.

Chapter **3**

Reflecting on ethical decision-making in therapy practice

Sally French

In the course of their daily work therapists are required to make numerous decisions. Some of these decisions are clinical in nature. The physiotherapist, for example, may decide that a client using crutches is safe to walk on his own, and an occupational therapist may conclude that a client has regained sufficient strength and balance to propel her wheelchair unaided. As well as making clinical decisions, however, therapists are also engaged in ethical decision-making. Indeed, clinical decisions frequently have an ethical component. If, for example, the client using crutches does not feel ready to walk on his own, or the person using a wheelchair prefers to rely on a helper, then an ethical issue will have arisen.

In the complex world in which we live, therapists are compelled to make ethical decisions every day. These decisions are not usually 'life or death' in nature and are less often aired in the media and the press as such topics as active euthanasia and abortion. This does not mean, however, that the issues confronted by therapists are mundane or trivial. If the client using a wheelchair is not given the help she feels she needs she may be too tired to engage in valued activities that maintain her happiness and self-esteem. Similarly, if the client using crutches is made to walk on his own before he feels he is ready to do so he may become nervous and distressed, which could have an adverse effect on his recovery. The fact that issues such as these are not discussed in a wider arena may mean that therapists lack exposure to differing perspectives that might help to guide their thinking and actions. None of this is to imply, however, that therapists are uninvolved in ethical decisions that may be thought more serious. They may, for example, be party to decisions involving the withdrawing of treatment from a dying person (passive euthanasia) or in following 'not for resuscitation' orders. Setting the scene, 'in context', then, this chapter turns to therapy as impacting on people's lives and the dilemmas this poses for therapists.

WHAT DO WE MEAN BY ETHICS?

Eby states that ethics:

> . . . is that branch of philosophy that is concerned with the systematic study of human values and the principles and methods of distinguishing right from wrong and good from bad. (2000, p. 120)

Similarly, Edge & Randall Groves define ethics as:

> ...that part of philosophy that deals with systematic approaches to questions of morality. It provides the intellectual framework that allows us to analyse and make decisions in regard to moral choices. (1999, p. 49)

The term 'ethics' is often used interchangeably with 'morals', but Sim (1997a) points out a subtle distinction in the use of these concepts. A person is said to be immoral if his or her behaviour goes against moral standards in a general sense. Unethical behaviour, on the other hand, violates a specific code of moral behaviour that is usually associated with a particular role. It might be considered immoral, for example, to buy your friend's fiancée expensive gifts, but it would be considered unethical for a therapist to do so for a client. Whether or not behaviour is considered 'moral' or 'immoral', 'ethical' or 'unethical', however, depends on the ideas, beliefs and assumptions we hold about our society and ourselves. These change over time and across cultures and there is always a diverse range of opinion (Edge & Randall Groves 1999). For example, 50 years ago divorce was a cause of disgrace and shame, whereas today it is considered by most a 'normal', if regrettable, part of modern life and by a few as being positively advantageous. Pahl, for example, states:

> Don't see divorce statistics and the growth of lone parent households as indicators of a lack of social cohesion. Rather see how friendships and the solidarity of single mothers are creating new, better and more equal bonds in society. (1995, pp. 21–22)

With regard to clinical practice an ethical issue that has changed considerably over the last 50 years has been that of telling the truth to clients. In the past, a paternalistic stance was usually taken that attempted to shield people from bad news such as terminal illness (and, no doubt, shielded health professionals from confronting difficult issues). It is now generally agreed that clients have the right to know, and that ignorance and uncertainty can give rise to distress that far surpasses 'the truth' if it is given in a sensitive and compassionate way. The issue of truth telling does, however, remain a source of ethical conflict.

There is, then, a lack of consensus about what constitutes moral and immoral, ethical and unethical behaviour. This applies as much to health care as any other area of life where there is far less public and professional moral consensus than there was in the past. Because of this diversity of opinion it is generally agreed that when important decisions are made within society, concerning genetic engineering, for example, that the decision-makers should come from varied social backgrounds. Moral authority cannot be based on professional expertise.

> **Reflections**
>
> With a colleague write down some areas of life where moral thinking has changed from your grandparents' generation to your own. What influences brought about these changes and how far are they contested today?

Health-care ethics refers to the application of ethical principles to health care. It is important to remember that ethics is 'applied' to health care rather than emanating from it. Although the processes of clinical and ethical decision-making are quite similar, it does not mean that because a decision is right clinically it is necessarily right ethically. A physiotherapist may, from his or her knowledge of human anatomy and physiology, believe that a client needs to exercise following a fractured ankle. If, however, the client refuses on the grounds that a permanently stiffened ankle is preferable to the pain and effort involved in mobilizing it, then to force her or him to exercise could be regarded as ethically unsound. As Sim states:

> What may seem an appropriate decision on clinical grounds may be morally objectionable and, conversely, what may seem a dubious decision purely in terms of clinical judgement, may have much to recommend it as a moral course of action. (1997b, p. 323)

Ethical reasoning in health care is not an 'armchair' activity but is concerned with developing the skills of reflection, analysis and logic in order to take appropriate action. This is sometimes referred to as 'practical ethics' or 'applied ethics'. As Kasar & Nelson Clark state:

> As a health care practitioner, you will be able to recognise ethical dilemmas, apply problem solving techniques, and come to a decision and then act in a way that you believe to be ethical and professional. (2000, p. 11)

We shall now consider various approaches to ethical decision-making.

The principles approach (deontology)

Deontology is taken from the Greek work for duty. With this approach fundamental principles are used to guide ethical decision-making. These principles include:

1. Respect for the person – this principle dictates that people should be treated with dignity and valued for their own worth and uniqueness. People should never be used for somebody else's ends as, for example, in research or as a means of educating student therapists.
2. Respect for autonomy – this principle dictates that people should be free to make their own choices unfettered by duress, deceit, coercion or constraint. We can violate someone's autonomy by restricting their freedom, or by

withholding or distorting information. This principle can require the enhancement as well as the preservation of autonomy. The violation of this principle 'for someone's own good' is known as paternalism.

3. Beneficence – this principle dictates that we should strive to do good, that we should '. . . act in ways that promote the welfare of other people' (Munson 1996, p. 34).

4. Non-maleficence – this principle dictates that we should avoid doing harm. Non-malificence means that therapists should neither intentionally harm their clients nor cause unintentional harm through carelessness.

5. Justice – this principle dictates that we should treat people fairly. According to this principle people should be treated in the same way unless there are relevant differences among them. It may be considered just, for example, for people to wait in a bus queue on a 'first come, first served' basis. If, however, a person in the queue is feeling unwell and needs to get home it may be considered unjust to make her wait her turn in the queue. This principle can, similarly, be applied to therapy waiting lists.

Secondary principles are derived from primary principles. For example, the secondary principle of telling the truth can be derived from the primary principles of autonomy and beneficence, although it may also be considered that distorting the truth is in the person's best interests in some situations (Rumbold 2000). Similarly, the secondary principles of confidentiality, fidelity and privacy, may be derived from the primary principles of non-maleficence and respect for the person. Ethical principles thus guide our actions.

Primary principles often conflict, in which case an attempt must be made to decide which one is weightier in the given circumstances.

Reflections

Consider the following hypothetical situation. Sarah, who has moderate learning difficulties, has recently been involved in a road traffic accident and, as a consequence, has a stiff and painful knee. Although she is keen on swimming, horse-riding and other sports, Sarah will not co-operate with Jackie, the physiotherapist, to bend her knee and become more mobile. Jackie is reluctant to coerce her and yet she is aware that Sarah derives a great deal of satisfaction, self-esteem and dignity from her sporting activities.

The principle of beneficence dictates that Jackie should carry out the treatment on Sarah's knee as this is for Sarah's own good. This, however, conflicts with the principle of respect for autonomy, which dictates that people have the right to choose for themselves even if they make unwise choices. Sarah has not given her consent to be treated by Jackie, so to force treatment upon her could be regarded as a paternalistic act that would violate Sarah's freedom and independence.

(Continued)

Reflections — continued

Ethical decisions must be justified in the light of the particular situation. The decision, therefore, needs to be based on an accurate assessment of the facts. Jackie would need to be sure, for example, that Sarah's unwillingness to co-operate is not simply an expression of fear or a lack of understanding of the outcome. She also needs to be sure that Sarah is still interested in sport, she is not unduly depressed or anxious, and pain or distress is not distorting her judgement. It is a mistake to think that people are necessarily irrational because they are experiencing symptoms, but if pain is a problem for Sarah Jackie could give a pain-relieving treatment, such as heat or massage, before commencing Sarah's exercises.

By checking out these factors Jackie is demonstrating respect for Sarah's autonomy far more than she would be by simply withdrawing treatment. If Sarah's behaviour is significantly influenced by any of these factors basing action on the 'respect for autonomy' principle would be flawed. It would also be unethical to allow Sarah to make the decision to refuse treatment without attempting to encourage her and give her information – that is, Sarah's refusal to have treatment must be fully informed. Nevertheless, the dividing line between persuasion and coercion is fine, especially in the context of an unequal relationship. The situation is also complicated by Sarah's learning difficulties. Jackie may consider, for instance, that Sarah is incapable of giving her informed consent and that it is justifiable for her to gain the consent of a parent or carer.

A further issue that complicates Jackie's position with regard to this ethical dilemma is that her values may conflict with those of her profession and other people in Sarah's life such as her parents or carers. Whereas Jackie may come to the conclusion that Sarah is an adult who knows her own mind, her manager may feel it is Jackie's role and duty as a physiotherapist to mobilize Sarah's knee. Sarah's carers, on the other hand, may feel unjustly served if Sarah's knee remains untreated because of the extra care that they may feel obliged to give. As well as being ethically accountable, therefore, Jackie is accountable to her managers, her professional body, to Sarah and to Sarah's carers. She may also be accountable legally for assault, if she forces physical treatment on Sarah against her will, or neglect if she fails in her duty as a physiotherapist.

Ethics is frequently intertwined with the law but is not the same. Not everything that is regarded as immoral is illegal and the law, though based on principles of justice, may be regarded as unjust. Kasar & Nelson Clark state that:

> Laws tell us what we shouldn't do and are based on rules that if violated are subject to legal sanctions. Ethics gives us standards to live by and guide our professional conduct. (2000, p. 14)

Some laws, for example the 1993 Mental Health Act, override moral considerations by allowing medical treatment to be carried out against the person's will.

It can be seen from the example of Sarah and Jackie that ethical decision-making is a highly complex affair and not a mere matter of opinion.

Consequentialism

In this approach to ethical decision-making the consequences of an action, which should not be harmful to the person, are more important than ethical principles. Let us take the case of a man who is terminally ill in hospital and has only a few days to live. During that time a catastrophic fire occurs at his house and destroys a large collection of valuable books that he has left in his will for his grandson. The deontologist may believe that the man's autonomy should be respected and that he should be told of the event so that he can decide for himself what to do. The consequentialist, on the other hand, may come to the conclusion that the man has enough problems to deal with already and that nothing will be gained by relating this news. He may, however, agree with the deontologist that the man should be told but the rationale for arriving at that decision will be different. He may decide, for example, that the losses incurred by the man's grandson, and his family, if he is left nothing in the will, outweigh consideration for the client himself. Deontologists uphold ethical principles (respect for autonomy in this example), whereas consequentialists are prepared to break ethical principles if it leads to a good outcome. Jackie, the physiotherapist in the example above, may, using a consequentialist analysis, conclude that to leave Sarah with a stiff and painful knee would damage her lifestyle as well as impede on the lives of her parents and carers. This judgement would override the principles of 'respect for the person' and 'respect for autonomy'.

One form of consequentialism is utilitarianism where the goal of morality can be identified as 'the greatest happiness to the greatest number'. The manager of a speech and language therapy department may conclude, for example, that it is better for each therapist to treat 10 people with mild aphasia in a day than 5 people with severe aphasia because in that way the greatest number of people will benefit. This principle does, of course, conflict with the principle of justice which, if followed, may arrive at the conclusion that those most in need should be given priority by the therapists.

The issue of how health and social care should be distributed is never far from the headlines and a utilitarian stance is often evident and disputed. Following the post-war welfare settlement, for example, the specific needs of individuals, such as people from ethnic minorities and disabled people, were neglected in favour of white men of working age (Langan 1998a, p. 8). In the 1990s, when the drive to curb spending on health- and social-care services was high on the government's agenda, there were various prominent cases in the newspapers, such as that in 1995 of Jaymee Bowen. He was a child with leukaemia who was refused further treatment ostensibly on the grounds of cost. An individual person may thus require an expensive treatment but be denied it on the grounds that it is not in the interests of the community to spend so much on one person or a particular group of people such as those who are old. In recent years such discussions have occurred over the chemical treatment of multiple sclerosis, AIDS and impotence.

Quasi-scientific measures have been applied to individuals in order to prioritize health- and social-care services from a utilitarian perspective (Beauchamp & Childress 2001). One of these is the quality-adjusted life years (QALY) measure, which attempts to provide an objective estimate of the costs and benefits of medical intervention. The basic measure is 1 year of healthy life as a result of medical treatment, multiplied by an assessment of the quality of life on a scale from 0 to 10. The cost per QALY can then be measured and those with the lowest costs are given priority. Ethical problems with this measure can immediately be seen. Who is to assess the quality of a person's life? Is it justifiable to discriminate against people who need expensive or long-term treatment? Using this measure it is likely that disabled people and people with serious illnesses would come low in the hierarchy for service provision (Langan 1998b), even though they have articulated serious flaws in the argument that their lives are necessarily of less quality than those of non-disabled people (French & Swain 2002). This is illustrated in the following quotations:

> I cannot wish that I had never contracted ME, because it has made me a different person, a person I am glad to be, would not want to have missed being, and could not relinquish even if I were cured. (Wendell 1996, p. 83)

> I do not wish for a cure for Asperger's syndrome. What I wish for is a cure for the common ill that pervades too many lives, the ill that makes people compare themselves to a normal that is measured in terms of perfect and absolute standards, most of which are impossible for anyone to reach. (Holliday-Willey 1999, p. 96)

Cain reminds health-care workers that:

> . . . if the patient's own perspective is given weight, bias and subjectivity in relation to quality of life judgements can be countered by the patient's own valuation of his or her life; and judgements based on the patient's condition can be made morally more secure if the patient's viewpoint is sought. (2002, p. 303)

Virtues approach

A further approach to ethics is to emphasize the characteristics of people who make ethical decisions. With this approach it is thought important for such people to possess the personality traits of courage, wisdom, sensitivity, compassion, and empathy in order to be capable of making sound ethical judgements. Kasar & Nelson Clark believe that:

We each have our own personal ethics that are shaped by religious beliefs, cultural heritage, family values, moral teaching, education and life experiences. (2000, p. 12)

By definition it can be argued that the therapist–client relationship is based on trust, which implies that therapists need to be honest and willing to exercise discretion when dealing with sensitive information. Sim is of the opinion that ' . . . moral virtue plays an important part both in the initial recognition of a moral problem and in the pursuit of action which has been identified as morally appropriate' (1997b, p. 327). It is certainly the case that evidence of traits such as empathy and compassion are valued in candidates for the health-care professions (French 2001). Sim cautions, however, that:

An uncritical focus on the cultivation of motives, virtues and character traits, to the exclusion of rigorous analysis of specific actions and their justification, may lead to a superficial and facile assumption that all that matters in health care is to be the 'right' sort of person. (1997a, p. 32)

Good intentions can certainly thwart creativity, violate autonomy and lead to the wrong action. To give a personal example, a few weeks ago I arrived at my office at work to discover a new telephone with very large numbers. This had been bought for me with some money left over in the departmental budget. Although I am visually impaired, and do use 'special' equipment, I did not ask for an adapted telephone and I certainly do not need one. The telephone is, in fact, a hindrance, as it is too big to allow me to place my hand over the keys and dial without looking, which I used to do. This example, though infuriating to me, is trivial compared with the experiences of many disabled people who have been at the receiving end of 'benevolent' action as the following examples illustrate:

I couldn't see the point of all those agonizing exercises. I was never very good at accepting the fact that things I didn't like could be 'good for me' and the physiotherapist managed to do a really good job of making me a conscientious objector for life. (Begum 1994, p. 48)

For young people the disadvantages of medical treatment need to be weighted against the possible advantages. Children are not usually asked if they want speech therapy, physiotherapy, orthopaedic surgery, hospitalisation, drugs or cumbersome and ugly 'aids and appliances'. We are not asked whether we want to be put on daily regimes or programmes which use hours of precious play-time. All these things are just imposed on us with the assumption that we share our parents' or therapists' desire for us to be more 'normal' at all costs. We are not even consulted as adults as to whether we think those things had been necessary or useful. (Mason & Rieser 1992, p. 82)

I hated learning speech – hated it – I felt so stupid having to repeat the s,s,s. . . . Every time I got it wrong. I had to do it all over again and I was asking myself 'Why do I have to keep going over and over it, I don't

> **Reflections**
>
> With a colleague who you trust discuss a difficult ethical dilemma that you have faced. Were you happy with the way the dilemma was resolved? If not, why not? What factors influenced your decision? Would you act in the same way if a similar dilemma arose again?

understand what it all means!' . . . It was just so stupid, a waste of time when I could have been learning more important things. (Corker 1996, p. 92)

Barnitt (2000) considers the virtues approach in the context of broad social and political factors. She believes that the virtues therapists extol may be the product of a patriarchal society in which women are expected to show care and compassion rather than more radical patterns of thought and behaviour. Thus rather than being within the person, virtues may be subject to outside influences and pressures. In her research with 16 occupational therapists and physiotherapists, Barnitt found that they were not always free to make their own decisions. She states:

In a perfect world, a therapist would decide which decision or course of action was best or most moral, and then implement it. In practice therapists are confronted with many situations where this is not possible, for example providing mobility or independence aids when there are resource shortages. Hard decisions have to be made about who is most deserving, and the therapist has to cope with criticism or formal complaints from those who have gone without. (2000, p. 105)

The therapists in this research spoke of loss of social support if they went against colleagues' expectations. They also experienced guilt and anxiety if they thought their actions left clients at risk. The therapists were motivated to maintain their own mental health and self-esteem as well as working in the interests of clients which, in itself, created conflict and anxiety. Those who were unsupported in assisting a client were left feeling angry and frustrated whereas those whose decision ran counter to their own values were left with feelings of helplessness. It can be seen that prudence, or the pursuit of self-interest, may enter into ethical decision-making. Very often there is no conflict as the client's and the therapist's interests are in accord, for example when giving informed consent. In extreme situations, when dealing with violent clients, for example, professionals may be relieved of their normal moral obligations in order to protect themselves.

Feminist approach

Central to the feminist approach to ethics are issues of male power and female subordination (Eby 2000). A reliance on ethical principles to guide action is regarded as limiting and inadequate and there is a far greater concern to analyze wide contextual factors, particularly with regard to patriarchy (Sherwin 2002). Gilligan (1982) noticed a difference in the way boys and men, and girls and women examined moral issues: whereas males searched out moral rules, females were more concerned with the relationships among those involved than with abstract ethical principles. Beauchamp & Childress assert that feminist accounts:

> . . . maintain that 'oppressive socialisation and oppressive social relationships' can impair autonomy, for instance, through forming an agent's desires, beliefs, emotions and attitudes, through thwarting the development of the capacities and competences essential for autonomy, and through various restrictions and limitations on the range of options for action. (2001, p. 61)

Although feminists are cautious in adopting gender-specific patterns of moral reasoning, their focus is on the relationships between the various agents and the narrative and contextual detail of each situation. Sherwin states that:

> Feminist ethics requires that any evaluation of moral considerations attend to the power relations that structure the relevant interactions. Political analyses of the unequal power between women and men, of white people and people of color, of First World and Third World people, of the rich and the poor, of the healthy and disabled and so forth are central to feminist ethics. To date that sort of analysis has been almost entirely absent from the literature of mainstream medical ethics although the institutions in which health care is provided are deeply implicated in the maintenance of structures of oppression. (2002, p. 27)

From the feminist viewpoint, then, there is little point in analyzing ethical issues unless consideration is taken of the power relationships that exist between, for example, therapists and clients, doctors and therapists, disabled and non-disabled people, and old and young people. What may seem, on the surface, to be an act of compassion between a male doctor and a female patient, or a non-disabled therapist and a disabled client may, when the relationships are analyzed, be interpreted as paternalistic or discriminatory.

Reflections

Write down any instances in your life where you have, on the surface, been treated with concern by health- and social-care professionals (or others in authority), but where you have felt an undercurrent of inequality and an imbalance of power. This may relate, for instance, to sexism, ageism, racism, homophobia or disablism. Are there any situations in your practice as a therapist where this kind of dynamic has operated with your clients? With a trusted colleague or client discuss the ways in which imbalances of power may be reduced in your practice as a therapist.

ETHICAL CODES AND GUIDELINES

Ethical codes and guidelines have been produced by the Chartered Society of Physiotherapy, the College of Occupational Therapists, and the College of Speech and Language Therapists. Such codes can assist with decision-making and also give guidance on duties, responsibilities and appropriate standards of behaviour. They can be used as a point of reference when disciplinary action is taken and may, therefore, afford some degree of protection for clients. As Sim states:

> . . . an ethical code is a consensus document. It represents the outcome of careful deliberation, by representatives of the profession as a whole as to the sort of conduct that is required from individual practitioners. As such it seeks to highlight the fundamental principles upon which one's professional life . . . should be conducted and to alert one to possible dilemmas and areas of conflict. (1997b, p. 329)

Clearly, the guidance offered by professional codes of conduct is broad and general and may not help the therapist who is grappling with a particular ethical dilemma. Indeed, professional codes may impede analysis and absolve the therapist of responsibility. Sim states:

> There is a danger that its codified nature, and the rather definitive terms in which it is expressed, may encourage the practitioner to think that 'the job has been done' and that further reflection on the issue concerned is redundant. As a result, decisions on ethical questions may become ineffective and stereotyped. (1997b, p. 334)

Barnitt (2000) found that very few therapists either read or use ethical guidelines.

Professional codes of conduct have a tendency to mix genuinely moral issues, about treating clients with respect, for example with issues that are more concerned with professional image and etiquette. Clark states that:

> Professional ethics comprise the more or less formalised principles, rules, conventions and customary practices that inform professionals' treatment of their clients, each other, and their relations to society at large. (2000, p. 272)

The Chartered Society of Physiotherapy's Revised Rules of professional conduct (1996), for example, requires physiotherapists to avoid criticizing other professionals and restraint when advertising their services. It also requires physiotherapists to behave in a way that will 'reflect credit on the profession'. As Homan remarks ' . . . ethical principles are established on the basis of a considerable measure of professional self-interest' (1991, p. 3). As noted earlier in this chapter, therapists may be required to act on behalf of various parties and failing to abide by hospital or professional policy may lead them into considerable trouble even if the policy is flawed on ethical grounds. Criticizing colleagues, even though there are sound ethical grounds for doing so, may have similar consequences and is 'high-risk, often lonely and rarely appreciated' (Edge & Randall Groves 1999, p. 95). 'Whistle-blowers' have, however, been given more protection in recent years (Brown 1999).

ETHICAL DECISION-MAKING

Sound ethical decision-making is dependent on honest, open communication with clients where their ideas, needs and aspirations are explored and respected. The unequal balance of power between therapists and their clients makes moral awareness particularly important. What may be the best course of action for one person may be calamitous for another and it is only by understanding the particular person concerned, and thinking through his or her situation carefully and logically, that the best solution will be found. We have already noted, however, that ethical considerations sometimes go beyond the individual person involved.

It is probably true to say that there are multiple perspectives that can be brought to bear on any problem and, despite the confusion that this may bring, it can also lead to creative new ideas. Ethical decision-making is a social act that can only be achieved by listening carefully and collaborating with the client to reach the best possible solution. Talking of cultural issues, Edge & Randall Groves state:

> It is important for providers to be sensitive to these differences among our patient population as they affect how willing the patient is to comply with our regimes or even whether the patient is willing to risk entry with our strange system. (1999, p. 250)

Wider discussion of ethical problems and issues with colleagues is also important in the development of ethical awareness and decision-making.

Ethical decisions are based on values and as we do not all have the same values ethical conflicts will always arise. Ethical decision-making cannot, therefore, be a precise affair and it may be necessary to weigh values and principles against each other in order to reach a decision. Eby points out, however, that ethical decision-making is logical and goes through the stages of gathering information, identifying the problem, seeking out solutions, choosing a solution and evaluating the decision. She believes that:

> One of the fundamental goals of the study of ethics is to help practitioners to develop practical reflective skills that can be used on a day to day basis to consolidate and reinforce ethical awareness and analysis . . . using an understanding of the various philosophical approaches to ethics and some sort of decision making process can enhance individuals' ability to work through their thinking on these issues and contribute to the decision making process. (2000, p. 138)

Thus ethical principles, though essentially subjective and never pure, can, nonetheless, be logically applied where the decision that is made is linked to moral principles or a philosophical position. The decision-making process and the decision itself need to be justified and based on an accurate assessment of the situation. As Sim states:

> ... the demands of ethical decision making are very similar to such processes as clinical diagnosis and treatment planning. In both cases there is a need for logical thought processes and close attention to the specific facts of the case in question followed by the formulation of a systematic plan of action. (1997b, p. 329)

Reflections

Read the following hypothetical case study of Samantha (a client) and Rob (an occupational therapist) and with one or more of your colleagues consider the ethical dilemmas posed. With reference to various ethical principles, explain systematically and logically what action should be taken.

> Samantha is attending occupational therapy following a fracture to her shoulder. After several treatment sessions she confides in the occupational therapist, Rob, that the medical history she gave him was false and that she sustained the fracture from Luke, her husband, following a row over money. She tells Rob that she does not want anyone else to know about what happened and that she does not want him to amend anything in her medical record. Rob asks Samantha if it has ever happened before and she says that it has but is adamant that she can handle the situation and does not want anyone else involved. Later in the session she tells Rob that she is worried about the effect the violence is having on her two children, Celia who is eight and Paul who is three, but does not believe anyone can help her. Rob asks if Luke has ever been violent towards the children and Samantha assures him that this has never happened and that she cannot imagine it ever will. Samantha tells Rob that the fault lies entirely with her because Luke has a low paid job and she spends too much money. She feels that the problem and the solution lie entirely in her own hands.

This extract contains various problems which need to be considered by Rob. First, there is Samantha who has sustained a serious injury from Luke who has been violent towards her. Second, there is the possible adverse effect the violence may be having on Samantha's children. Finally, there is the issue of whether or not to correct the false medical record.

Rob may decide not to disclose the information Samantha has given him. This can be justified on the grounds of 'respect for the person' and 'respect for autonomy'. From his professional relationship with Samantha, Rob may conclude that she is a rational person who must make her own decisions in this sensitive area of her life. He is acutely aware of the importance of trust and confidentiality in the client–therapist relationship and regards discretion and

(Continued)

Reflections — continued

the safeguard of Samantha's privacy as a major aspect of his professional role. He considers the ethical principle of non-maleficence and concludes that he may do more harm than good by breaking Samantha's confidence and involving other people. Rob is concerned about Samantha's children but believes, from what Samantha has said, that they are not in danger of physical abuse. He feels uneasy about leaving the medical record unamended as he is aware that it is bad practice and could have legal implications. He decides to place moral duties above legal ones and is prepared to take any consequences that arise. As he is seeing Samantha twice a week he decides to encourage her to talk more about her life and her problems so that he can gain a fuller understanding and, in time, encourage her to seek the help she needs.

An alternative scenario may be that after hearing Samantha's story Rob feels that she is in serious danger from Luke and that a social worker and the police should be involved. He knows from the nature of the fracture that the violence towards Samantha was extreme and cannot be justified in any way. He takes a consequentialist approach believing that more harm will come to Samantha and her children if he does nothing than if he breaks her confidence. This approach also overrides any considerations he has about the nature of his role as an occupational therapist or the client–therapist relationship. He knows that Samantha is rational, but believes that his actions are in her best interest and those of her children (the principle of beneficence) even though they may be considered paternalistic. On consequentialist grounds Rob is also of the opinion that correct medical records are vital for the welfare of clients and society as a whole. He intends, however, to talk the whole matter over carefully with his manager and the social worker in his team before taking any action.

Both of these examples, though reaching opposite conclusion, link the dilemmas Rob is facing with ethical theories and principles. Neither solution is 'right' or 'wrong', in an absolute sense, and in a real-life situation there may have been other factors to guide Rob's decision.

In undertaking this exercise you may have reached other conclusions. In the first scenario, for instance, Rob may have deduced that to break Samantha's confidence would be detrimental on consequentialist grounds because clients would then trust therapists less with negative implications for rehabilitation overall. In the second example he may have highlighted utilitarianism in consideration of Samantha's children. The important thing is that you used all available evidence from the extract and that your decision was systematic and logical taking ethical principles and moral theory into account. In reality, ethical decision-making is frequently an ongoing process. As you learn more and more about a client, what may first seem an ideal solution may become less appropriate.

CONCLUSION

Ethical issues permeate every aspect of the therapist's work including giving information, consultation, physical contact, and allocating time and resources. Ethical decision-making is equally as important as clinical decision-making in therapy practice. It is part of the role of every therapist to make ethical decisions carefully in the light of each particular case and to justify the course of action taken if required. Although there are no definitive answers to ethical dilemmas, ethical decision-making is always more than personal opinion or 'common sense'.

PART 2

In theory and principle

Part 2 turns to concepts and theories that cast light on enabling relationships. There is a whole array of relevant theories. We are not attempting here, however, to present a comprehensive summary of the theories, but rather provide foundations to help further your reflections on enabling relationships. It is important to note that no one formal theory underpins the approach within this book and key concepts provide the starting points to focus the discussions. In Chapter 4, John Swain and Sally French begin by exploring concepts of inequality, particularly economic and health inequalities. They then turn to concepts of power, theories of power, in relations between groups of people and in interpersonal relationships, touching on Weber's and Foucault's ideas. This provides a basis for looking at ways of understanding discrimination and oppression. Karen Parry then turns the focus to theories of social change, beginning with the key concepts of empowerment and emancipation. She then critiques reductionist and deterministic viewpoints. Karen briefly summarizes theories of feminism, symbolic interactionism and existential psychology as offering ways of trying out new narratives by which to construct the relationship between therapists and clients. To conclude Part 2, John Swain attempts to bridge the gap between theory and therapy practice by providing a framework of principles for enabling relationships, critical reflection, and empowerment and emancipatory practice. He presents a tentative model for a working alliance: to enable people to develop their own potential; to enable people to have a voice and to be heard; to respect the diversity of people's aspirations and values; and to challenge unequal power relations between people.

Chapter **4**

Understanding inequality and power

John Swain and Sally French

What does the word inequality mean to you? To set the scene, consider Carol's story:

> I want to get more money. I'd like to get £8.
> I get £3.50 for work in the mornings in the centre.
> Before she left, Mrs James said we'd get more money, but we have not had it yet.
> Sometimes I get money at the hostel for helping out with the cleaning. My aunt buys my clothes. I use my money to buy the *Radio* and *TV Times*. I save £2, and spend it at the club on a Saturday night. *Carol.*
> (Atkinson & Williams 1990, p. 138)

Carol's story is a reflection of the unequal distribution of wealth, privilege and power. It is a story of poverty. As we shall see in this chapter, the development of a global capitalist economy has seen ever sharper disparities between those at the top and those at the bottom of social hierarchies in recent

---

Reflections

List the main factors that might be significantly associated with inequality between people. What questions might be raised in understanding Carol's circumstances?

We would suggest the following:

1. Economics – What are Carol's financial resources and what are the possibilities of increasing her economic status?
2. Gender – To what extent is Carol's gender significant in her opportunities and access to resources?
3. Race/ethnicity – Is Carol a member of an ethnic minority?
4. Age – Is Carol's age relevant in understanding her financial resources?
5. Disability – Is disability a significant factor in Carol's lack of financial resources?

years. The losers in the current processes of social and economic change include old people, ethnic minority members, disabled people and unemployed people. Social hierarchies are manifested and maintained in many ways, including racism, disablism, sexism, classism, homophobia and ageism. The losers are marginalized and excluded from the lifestyles and quality of life enjoyed by prosperous and elite groups.

Questions of inequality pervade understandings of identity, health and illness, the provision of human services. This chapter asks you to stand back from inequality, explore some of its manifestations in society, and find some ways of explaining inequalities. This takes us into the realms of concepts of ideology, oppression and discrimination. But let's begin with a parade!

Drawing on an original idea by Jan Penn, a Dutch economist, Mackintosh & Mooney (2000) (see also Hills 1995) graphically describe the unequal distribution of incomes in the UK as an 'income parade'. Imagine the total population of the UK, all 60 million, are lined up and rushed past you, and this parade of people takes just 1 hour from start to finish. Imagine too that the height of the people in the parade matches their household income, so that the greater the person's household income the taller he or she is. The average height of the people in the parade is 5 feet 8 inches and this is the height of the couples with an average household income (statistics taken from the early 1990s). So, here they come racing past, from the shortest (the poorest) to the tallest (the richest). After 3 minutes a single unemployed mother of two children passes by. She is living below income support level and is 1 foot 10 inches tall. Everyone who passes in the first 12 minutes has less than half the average income and so is less than 2 feet 10 inches tall. After 21 minutes the man passing by is a full-time vehicle exhaust fitter and his wife who is not in paid employment. They are 3 feet 9 inches tall. After half an hour, with half the population having gone past you, it may surprise you that the people passing are not of average height. They are only 4 feet 10 inches tall with a household income that is only 83% of the national average. When do people with an average household income pass by? Those of average height, with average income, do not pass you until 62% of the population have passed by, but to understand why this is we need to look to the end of the parade. After three-quarters of an hour the people are getting taller, about 6 feet 10 inches now, but it is not until the last 10 minutes that the height of the people passing really begins to grow. With 3 minutes left the couple passing are 11 feet 11 inches tall. They are in their late 50s and their children have left home. He is a self-employed freelance journalist and she is a part-time manager of an old people's day centre. In the last minute a company chief executive and his wife, who is not in paid employment, pass by. They are both at least 60 feet tall. It is in the last seconds that the real giants arrive, people whose heights can be measured in miles, the richest being at least 4 miles tall. We think this graphically illustrates economic inequality, from being less than 2 feet tall to having your head in the clouds. Evidence also suggests that this gap is widening. Definitions of poverty are disputed. A common measure, however, is a household income at, or below, half the national average (those passing by in the income parade for the first 12 minutes). In the UK the number of people living in poverty rose from 5 million to 13.9 million in the years between 1979 and 1991–2. (The information in this section is taken from Mackintosh & Mooney 2000, pp. 87–89, 92.)

Poverty, however it is defined, is not simply a matter of lack of financial resources as in the income parade. There are, as Thompson suggests, significant social implications in terms of:

- psychological well-being, particularly in relation to self-esteem
- social relations – low income groups can be marginalized or excluded in certain social situations
- insecurity – economic deprivation can make it difficult, if not impossible, to plan ahead or develop a 'lifeplan'
- access to resources and services – for example health and education. (1998, p. 91)

So what about the 'client parade' – that is, the line up of clients that pass through therapy? What would the parade of clients who passed through therapy last year look like? Perhaps you might like to imagine them passing by you in an hour-long parade! The statistics are not available, though it is highly unlikely that the client parade is a simple reflection, or random sample, from the income parade. One important factor in the client parade, is the distribution of health problems, and it is to inequalities and health that we turn next.

INEQUALITIES AND HEALTH

To take our exploration of inequalities into the field of health we need first to consider what we mean by 'health'. Health is a complex concept that encompasses physical, psychological and social well-being. It is not, therefore, merely concerned with the absence of disease and illness, but permeates the whole of life (Benzeval et al. 1995a). This is reflected in the book *Meeting the Health Needs of People Who Have a Learning Disability* (Thompson & Pickering 2001), which contains chapters on self-concept, meaningful occupation and life transitions. As Souza & Ramcharan state:

> Being healthy and staying healthy happens when you have a meaning to your life. It is no good asking people to look after themselves if they have no reason to do so. Having meaning to your life means having a reason to keep fit and healthy such as going to work, participating in leisure and seeing friends. (2001, pp. 174–175)

There are many influences on our physical, psychological and social health. Dahlgren & Whitehead (1991) depict these as layers piled on top of each other. At the bottom of the pile are biological factors over which we have limited, or no, control. These include our sex, age and the genes we inherit from our parents. Many diseases become more common as we grow older (for example cancer and cardiovascular disease), some diseases are specific to men or women (for example prostate and ovarian cancer), while others are genetic or congenital in origin (for example cystic fibrosis and congenital heart disease).

The second layer focuses on our personal behaviour. This includes whether or not we smoke cigarettes or eat too much, the amount of exercise we take and how well we attend to our health needs in the broadest sense. Most policy initiatives from government have focused on this layer where attempts have been made to change peoples' behaviour in order to improve their health (Jones 2000).

The next level concerns social and community influences. The people around us, including family members, neighbours and friends, can influence our health by giving meaning to our lives, and providing assistance and support in times of illness, difficulty and stress. Organizations such as the church and self-help groups may also be important. Conversely, these people can have a detrimental effect on our health, by neglect, abuse or failing to take account of our needs. Our behaviour may also be influenced, for good or ill, by peer pressure.

Living and working conditions comprise the next layer of influence. It is well known, for example, that the type of house in which we live and our environment at work can affect our health. Work pressure or noisy neighbours may cause depression and anxiety that can lead to physical ill health (Leon & Walt 2001), and physical hazards, such as dampness, poor architectural design and dangerous work practices, can cause disease and accidents. Much of the legislation passed by the Victorians improved people's health by tackling problems at this level. Various factory, housing and sanitation acts, for example, reduced the incidence of serious diseases, such as tuberculosis and typhoid, as well as improving the quality of people's lives generally (Gray 2001). Le Fanu (1999) claims that there was a 92% decline in tuberculosis before the introduction of curative drugs and similar evidence has been put forward by McKeown (1984) concerning many other life-threatening diseases, such as poliomyelitis and diphtheria.

The outermost layer affecting our health concerns general socio-economic, cultural and environmental conditions. This includes the economic state of the country, the level of employment, the tax system, the degree of environmental pollution and our attitudes, for example, towards women, ethnic minorities and disabled people. Increasingly, these factors are taking on an international dimension as globalization accelerates.

It is clear that these factors all interact and influence each other. If the economic state of the country is favourable, for example, people are likely to have more disposable income, which may improve their health by allowing them to buy good-quality food and obtain housing of a better standard, engage in leisure pursuits, give their children more opportunities and enjoy relaxing holidays to reduce stress. Similarly, if a person is attempting to give up drugs, success is more likely if community support is strong and if the government is willing to act by setting up and financing supportive policies. As Whitehead states:

If one health hazard or risk factor is focused upon, it is important to examine how it fits in with other layers of influence and whether it could be considered a primary cause or merely a symptom of a much larger problem represented in some other layer. (1995, p. 24)

Let's return to the income parade. Is health randomly distributed, i.e. can illness strike anyone at any time irrespective of their height in the income parade? As you might suspect, the answer is no, health is not randomly distributed. In most countries of the world there are large inequalities in health, with those of the lowest socio-economic status having the worst health. Certain groups within society, such as women, old people, people from ethnic minorities and disabled people, are also disadvantaged, partly because of their over-representation in the lower socio-economic groups. There are also regional variations in health status (French 1997a). Furthermore, in Britain, as in most countries of the Western world, these inequalities are increasing (Department of Health 2001). Benzeval et al. state that:

> It is one of the greatest contemporary social injustices that people who live in the most disadvantaged circumstances have more illness, more disability and shorter lives than those who are more affluent. In Britain death rates at most ages are two to three times higher among the growing number of disadvantaged people than they are for their better off counterparts. Most of the main causes of death contribute to these differences and together they can reduce life expectancy by as much as eight years. (1995b, p. 1)

These inequalities in health exist however socio-economic class is measured and at all stages of the life span.

Despite the various influences on our health, which were detailed above, the evidence overwhelmingly suggests that broad social factors concerning housing, income, educational level, employment and social integration are far more important than our individual behaviour or medical practice and advances. As Benzeval et al. state:

> The evidence shows quite convincingly that the more we increase our understanding of the determinants of health, the more inescapable is the conclusion that a person's health cannot be divorced from the social and economic environment in which they live and work. (1995b, p. 4)

Reflections

Think of a health-damaging behaviour that you, or someone close to you, have indulged in. What psychological and social factors influenced the behaviour? What purpose did the behaviour serve?

There is often a vicious circle in operation that can continue over generations. Benzeval et al. state:

> There is a body of evidence that poor socio-economic circumstances are highly correlated with low levels of educational attainment. In turn, the lack of educational qualifications increases the probability of unemployment and poverty in adulthood which are associated with poor health outcomes. (1995c, p. 127)

People of the lowest socio-economic status are at far higher risk, not only of physical illness and early death, but also of accidents, premature births, mental illness and suicide. Contrary to the popular image of the hard-working professional, it is those in boring, monotonous occupations, where there is excessive surveillance and little opportunity for control or creativity, that are under the most stress.

As mentioned above, most government initiatives to improve people's health in Britain have focused on strategies to change individual behaviour, often adopting a 'victim blaming' stance. People may be urged to diet or give up smoking and may be helped with counselling, self-help groups and stress-management programmes. It is now known, however, that our behaviour is largely determined by our social circumstances. If drug users are returned to the community without support following successful treatment, for example, they are likely to drift back to the their old way of life with the people they know and trust. Smoking, like most behaviours, is linked to social circumstances and people who are trying to give it up will often avoid situations, like in pubs, where they may be tempted or where peer pressure may be high. This is not to suggest that personal approaches are never beneficial. Personal empowerment, through assertiveness training for example, can be helpful, especially if it is linked with social support and social change.

It is a mistake to imagine that health-damaging behaviours are irrational. People in poverty may smoke or give children sweets in order to cope successfully with a difficult situation. Excessive alcohol consumption, smoking, over-eating and drug use may also be a way of containing difficult emotional and psychological problems. Despite the individualistic stance of most policies, the present government has taken some heed of the social determinant of health in, for example, attempting to improve education, housing and transport (Department of Health 1999).

There is no obvious correlation between health care and health status in any population; indeed, the health service has sometimes been referred to as an 'ill health' service as it tends to respond when the damage has been done. Benzeval et al. state:

> There is little evidence that variations in the quantity and quality of health services between advanced industrial countries make a substantial difference to crude measures of health such as national mortality rates . . . Levels of well-being and life expectancy are more closely related to the availability of decent social security, housing, employment and education than health care. (1995b, p. 96)

This is not to imply that inequalities in health and health-care facilities should be tolerated. Health care should be distributed in accordance with need. There is evidence, for example, that the up-take of immunization, birth control, antenatal care and screening is low among poor people. This is due to a range of factors that were summed up by Tudor Hart (1971) in his notion of the 'inverse care' law. People with low incomes find it harder to access health-care premises because of social isolation and lack of facilities such as a car. It is also the case that the areas in which they live tend to have poor facilities and that health professionals tend to give them less time and attention than people who are perceived to be culturally similar to themselves (French 1997b).

There are still many people in Britain who do not fully benefit from the facilities of the NHS. People from ethnic minorities are not well served (Atkin in press) nor people with learning difficulties (Shaughnessy & Cruse 2001).

This is due to a variety of factors that include poor communication, racism, disablism and lack of cultural sensitivity. Fox & Benzeval state:

> Access to health services cannot be taken for granted especially in the most disadvantaged communities. There is still much to be done to ensure that services are provided in appropriate locations, that user charges do not deter people from expressing legitimate needs and that cultural diversity is not ignored . . . people must be involved in helping to identify their own needs and services must be provided in ways that users themselves recognise as legitimate. (1995, p. 11)

Fox & Benzeval believe that an important role of the NHS should be to encourage social equity across all public departments and policies that have an impact on health. They state:

> Its first responsibility is to ensure greater equity of access to care by distributing resources in relation to needs and removing barriers that inhibit effective use of services. Secondly, all parts of the NHS have an obligation to promote a greater orientation towards equity and the development of healthy public policies both nationally and locally. (1995, p. 119)

The enactment of such a change would involve an increase in services such as outreach, the mobilization of self-help groups and community action and empowerment. At a broader level, it would necessitate involvement in areas such as housing, employment, education, leisure and community regeneration. Such a development would move therapists from their role as clinical practitioners dealing with the consequences of ill health, to the broader arena of health promotion and political activism.

Reflections

Think and talk about the possibilities and implications of such a change in role. Do you think this is a desirable change in role for therapists? What are the barriers to such a change? What are the main strengths in therapy practice that could be built on in effectively realising such a change?

UNDERSTANDING INEQUALITIES: POWER

The social sciences are awash with understandings of inequality; indeed, it could be said that the social sciences are founded on understanding inequality at its broadest, including individual differences, cultural differences and social hierarchies. How shall we approach this vast arena? How might this be of relevance to you as a therapist? The key is the concept(s) of power. The income and client parades are not just hierarchies of wealth, or household incomes, as we have seen in relation to health. The gulf between the rich and the poor, those who are miles high and those who are less than 2 feet tall, is one of 'social wealth', of choices, opportunities and access – or, in a word, power. Personal relationships are suffused with power, however it is conceived, and economics is only part of the complex picture. As will have become apparent in previous chapters, power is also inherent in therapist–client relationships. To engage with questions of enabling relationships is to engage with questions of power, both between therapist and client, and within the social worlds of which both are a part. In this chapter we explore some of the workings of power, then the constraints on people through oppression and discrimination. It is on the grounds of recognition and awareness of power imbalances that we turn in the next chapter to notions of empowerment and emancipation.

So what does power mean to you? What do you think of when you think of the term 'power'? It is, of course, a huge, diverse concept and your thinking could have taken you off in many different directions. It may have conjured, for instance, world power and perhaps the military might of the USA. Rather than being a parade of individuals, the income parade could be a parade of countries.

> The USA, EU and Japan make up a triad accounting for between two-thirds and three-quarters of all economic activity. Thus 85 per cent of the world's population are almost written out of any economic globalisation process. (Thompson 2000, p. 117)

Or perhaps you thought of the economic power of multi-national companies, such as McDonald's, or national politics, or legal power. Perhaps the word invokes power relations of class, race/ethnicity, gender and age, or the power relations of personal and professional relationships. The concept of power spans the whole gamut from the minutiae of everyday interactions to global structural power. It is not surprising, then, that in grappling to understand and explain power, social scientists have developed many different ways of thinking about it.

The notion of ideology is a useful starting point as, although the term is used in different ways it usually refers to commonly held beliefs about inequalities. An ideology is a set of ideas that systematically distort reality. It refers to 'sets of ideas, beliefs and assumptions in general and, more specifically, ... those that reflect existing power relations' (Thompson 1998, p. 20). Ideologies play an important role in the exercising of power. The power relations that characterize all of our social interactions are played out (among other ways) in the language we use to describe our lives. Dominant ideologies are sets of ideas that legitimate inequalities in different ways. They represent and strengthen the position of powerful groups and are shaped and maintained according to distributions of power (Dallos 1997). Ideologies conceal unacceptable aspects of reality; they give social status and aggrandize, and they make out that things that are neither natural nor necessary are actually both. Thinking back to the income parade, what are the commonly held beliefs about economic inequality? We are bombarded with messages that tell us that a hierarchy is natural, that it reflects natural capacity and individual merit. Notions of social necessity also legitimate inequalities, such as the belief that a hierarchy provides a ladder to climb and the motivation to succeed.

We turn next to two contrasting notions of how power might work in relationships. When you think of power, do your thoughts turn to force or coercion? Power can be seen as the capacity of one person to dominate another and something that is held and exercised by individuals, groups or institutions (or nation states) to directly secure their interests. This is the line of reasoning in Max Weber's theory of power (Weber 1978). As you read the following summary of Weber's ideas, think about how you might exercise power as a therapist, but think too about how power might be exercised over you. For Weber, power is:

> The probability that a person will be able to carry out his or her own will in the pursuit of goals of action, regardless of resistance. He defined 'domination' in a similar manner as the probability that a command would be obeyed by a given group of people. This definition has the following characteristics: (1) power is exercised by individuals and, therefore, involves choice, agency and intention; (2) power involves the notion of agency – that is, an individual achieving or bringing about goals that are desirable; (3) power is exercised over other individuals and may involve resistance and conflict; (4) power implies that there are differences in interests between the powerful and the powerless; and (5) power is negative, involving restrictions and deprivations for those subjected to domination (Abercrombie et al. 1994, p. 329).

For Weber, then, power is a hierarchical, top–down affair. Some people order and command while others obey but then direct the actions of others further down the ladder.

Returning to the income parade, clearly the taller you are the more power you exercise and, for Weber, social life is about inequality. He did not see inequality as necessarily economic, however. Though economic inequality frequently takes a leading part, it is only one form of inequality. Weber also thought that status groups were part of the picture. Status groups are differentiated by prestige – that is, the level of esteem in which people hold themselves and/or in which they are held by others. This idea of status groups reminds us of the well-known sketch in which John Cleese represents the upper-class, Ronnie Barker the middle-class and Ronnie Corbett the working-class. Like the income parade this is status by height. You may remember how they address each other: 'I look up to him because . . . ', 'I look down on him because . . . ' and, in the case of Ronnie Corbett, the shortest, 'I know my place'. We are reminded too of multi-professional groups we have experienced – with doctors, therapists, nurses, social workers – and clients. We are not suggesting it was as clear cut as in the comedy sketch, but certainly status clearly played a role in power relations.

'Party' is another element in Weber's analysis of power and inequality. It is a reflection of resistance and struggle in unequal power relations, and is the self-conscious organization for the pursuit of power. Ideas of resistance and resilience are crucial to the development of enabling relationships in therapy. Empowerment comes from people themselves and can be supported and facilitated but not given by the powerful to the powerless. We shall return to the notion of resistance.

As we have already indicated, this hierarchical notion is not the only view of power. You may have noted that hierarchies of power are not always what they seem. One person can ostensibly have power over another, but it is the supposedly less powerful person that is controlling the other, perhaps through more subtle manipulation. You may, for instance, know of families in which the children in subtle, and not so subtle, ways control the parents. Power may not always be negative. Think, for instance, of the power to oblige people to wear seat belts, power to prevent pollution, power to contest discrimination against any group within society. You might also think of power as a far more insidious affair that constrains relationships like a social mould. If so, you are thinking more along the lines of Foucault. He was interested in how power is exercised and its effects rather than who has power. From Foucault's viewpoint, the power within the establishment in which you work does not pass top – down; it is, rather, expressed through a matrix of organizational practices. This 'grid' of institutional practice induces and justifies certain courses of action, and denies and invalidates others. It may help to think about institutional discrimination, e.g. racism or disablism. This can be defined as:

> Unfair or unequal treatment of individuals or groups which is built into institutional organisations, policies, and practices at personal, environmental, and structural levels. (Swain et al. 1998, p. 5)

Reflections

Using Weber's ideas about power, consider your own situation as a therapist. First, think of yourself within hierarchies of power. Who has power over you? Do others restrict your choices, agency and intentions? Who do you have power over? Do you restrict the choices, agency and intentions of others? Second, what questions come to mind as you think about power in this way? How well does this way of thinking characterize your relationships as a therapist?

The power that is expressed through unequal treatment, then, is not in the hands of any one person but suffused through all the functioning and ways of working within the institution.

Foucault's ideas about power are complex and were developed throughout his writings. Power works on the basis of inducing and calling forth certain selective choices and closing down other possibilities:

> It incites, it induces, it seduces, it makes easier or more difficult; in the extreme it constrains or forbids absolutely; it is nevertheless always a way of acting upon an acting subject or acting subjects by virtue of their acting or being capable of action. (Foucault 1982, p. 220)

Language and, in particular, discourse are central. Power, knowledge and language are intimately interwoven. Ways of speaking, vocabularies, rules regulating what it is possible to say, who can say things, under what circumstances, and with what consequences create the matrix of power. Thus, the workings of power are internalized, and we comply with what seem to be self-evident truths.

Even in such a brief summary it is crucial to mention Foucault's ideas about resistance. From this viewpoint, wherever there is power there is resistance. They go hand in hand. The network, or matrix, of power relations is mirrored by a multiplicity of forms of resistance. Power, in this view, is not simply something that some have and use negatively over others who do not have power. Power is both constraining and enabling.

UNDERSTANDING THE DYNAMICS OF OPPRESSION

To draw this chapter to a close we return to the notion of oppression. It is a term that is clearly associated with the use of power and inequalities. Let's start by turning to a definition of what it means to 'oppress' taken from the *Oxford Dictionary*: 'govern tyrannically, keep under coercion, subject to continual cruelty or injustice.' You may have personal experiences that would illustrate such tyranny of one individual or group over another and, of course, history and present-day politics both nationally and internationally affords us with numerous examples. Yet it is a limited view of oppression. It is a value-laden term with connotations of the deliberate use of power by powerful people to restrict and control powerless people. This definition of what it means can conjure the idea that oppression is done by others to others, the oppressors to the oppressed, rather than being inherent within the unequal social relations within which we all live and all actively contribute to.

Oppression is multi-dimensional. Thompson focuses his influential work on discrimination:

> I shall therefore define discrimination as the process (or set of processes) by which people are allocated to particular social categories with an unequal distribution of rights, resources, opportunities and power. It is a process through which certain groups and individuals are disadvantaged and oppressed. (1998, p. 78)

Dominelli argues, however, that this 'emphasises only one element in the web of oppressive social relations' (2002, p. 4). As a basis for anti-oppressive theory and practice, she looks beyond the competitive terms that result in a winner and a loser. Dominelli seeks:

> A holistic framework that enables users to play a greater role in the design and delivery of the services they require and professionals to respond more appropriately to the agendas that they set. (2002, p. 5)

In this book we are also tentatively reaching for such a holistic framework for therapists wishing to establish enabling relationships in their work.

As we saw in Chapter 1, notions of oppression can also challenge ways of thinking that are grounded in binary social divisions. To take disability as an example: oppression cannot be understood solely within the relations between non-disabled and disabled people. This positions people in single categories, in this case disabled or non-disabled, and does not recognize the complex interplay of differences of age, race, religion, sexuality, gender and so on that is integral to the lives and identities of all disabled and non-disabled people. Again this can shift the emphasis to voices of those who experience oppression. Williams states:

> . . . breaking up analytic categories in this way . . . enables us to detach ourselves from the categories and meanings imposed by policy-makers, welfare managers . . . and to pursue what the categories of 'single mother', 'the old', 'the disabled', and so on, mean to those who inhabit them. (1996, p. 68)

Understandings of oppression can challenge the idea that oppressed people are the passive recipients of oppression. People resist and redefine their identity in positive terms. Black groups, women's groups, gay and lesbian groups, and organizations of disabled people are not passive recipients of oppression and discrimination, but have a long-standing history of political and cultural resistance. At its most radical, difference is not just recognized or espoused, but celebrated: 'Black is beautiful'; 'disability pride'. In relation to women's affirmation of female identity, Williams states:

> Not only did it turn the notion of women's difference from men on its head, it also proposed that the basis for women's political identity was not so much rooted in women's shared oppression by men but in women's shared identity as different from men. (1966, p. 67)

Once again the defining and dismantling of oppression is in the voices of those who experience oppression.

Thus, arguing from the multi-dimensional nature of oppression, from the challenging of binary oppositions and from the importance of resistance, understandings of the dynamics of oppression comes from experiences of oppression. Here is the starting point for enabling relationships in the framework developed through this book. Dalrymple & Burke take a similar stance as a foundation for anti-oppressive practice:

It is from the experiences of people who have been marginalised, who have had their rights denied or violated, that we can understand what is meant by oppression. (By listening to other people's experiences of oppression we are able to extend the parameters of what is possible [Lorde 1984]. It is the *listening* that is most important, as this provides us with the information that enables us to gain a fuller understanding of the issues. (1995, p. 15)

Reflections

Let's end this chapter with a poem as food for thought.

> oppression is not a choice
> or just the misfortune of the socially deprived
> no woman has ever escaped
> sexism like quiet rain
> constantly, softly seeping in
> until we all become saturated
> and it gently, ever so gently
> so we hardly notice
> does us terrible violence
> (Aspen 1983)

From your experience of therapy practice think of an example of the 'terrible violence' of oppression as experienced by a client.

1. Outline, from your viewpoint, the dynamics of oppression in this 'case'. Think broadly to include every aspect of social deprivation.
2. Outline what you think are the dynamics of oppression from the client's viewpoint. If you can, of course, draw on the client's expressed views and experiences.
3. In what ways might the client's views differ from your own?

Chapter 5

Understanding empowerment and emancipation

Karen Parry

In this chapter I will be looking at the theoretical foundations for enabling relationships in professional support, and the role of empowerment and emancipation within therapeutic practice. First, I would like to start by introducing myself. In many ways this is crucial to the chapter as it is about naming and defining, selecting characteristics about myself that may help you to locate me within your own structures of meaning. This will in turn impact upon how you perceive what is written and the validity this has for your practice. These issues are central to this chapter as this same process occurs in interactions with clients, as we base our understandings of them upon certain characteristics that have meaning for us. So, me. Professionally, I qualified as a teacher, dropped out of teaching and began as a care assistant within a short break home for disabled children, and worked my way up to take the opportunity to act as assistant officer in charge for a year. After 4 years within this establishment, I moved to a government-funded early-years project where I worked as volunteer co-ordinator, and, following a short spell here, I took a development post with the local Social Services Children with Disabilities Team. During this time I studied towards my PhD, finally completing it in December 2001.

This leads me on to saying something about myself personally. I have always been interested in issues of identity, self, being on the margins of mainstream society, and being critically aware of the constructed nature of categories presented as natural and innate. This interest underpinned my PhD and motivates the choices I make both professionally and personally. Collaborating on this book was one such decision.

Within this chapter, then, I will critique reductionist and deterministic viewpoints and go on to suggest three alternative perspectives that offer opportunities to think about the enabling relationship in new ways. These will be symbolic interactionism, feminism and existential psychology. No one of these theories is presented as superior or 'right', but instead they offer new ways of thinking about social interactions and working in a therapeutic role, and may provoke new ideas that can transform the ways in which we incorporate an empowering and emancipatory approach in practice. Each will offer ways of viewing personal lives, processes of interpersonal relationships and the nature of the social world, and will suggest ways in which to critically reflect on practice.

CONCEPTS OF EMPOWERMENT AND EMANCIPATION

While working in an early-years project in a so-called 'disadvantaged' area, I found some colleagues resisted the term empowerment when talking about work with parents, as they claimed this was patronizing and inherently disempowering. It was a heavily professionally driven project, with only minimal parental involvement. The government rhetoric for the underpinning philosophy of the project, however, was parental partnership with professionals. Thus, the issue had to be explicitly addressed. Within the project, the overriding understanding of the term empowerment was for the powerful professionals to share some of that power with the parents, but within tightly controlled boundaries, to only give them as much power as the experts believed they could handle. Of course giving this the label of empowerment was patronizing, as was the whole approach.

Thompson (1993) argues that to enable a person to become more empowered, one has to shift from an approach of charity and compassion to one of rights and advocacy, and this was the key to the difficulty within this project. A small group of workers within the project developed a parents' committee, which aimed to create a space in which people could become empowered, taking control of decisions, rather than accepting what was given to them in the name of empowerment. The result was mixed. It was a difficult group to work with, as individuals grappled with responsibilities they had never previously experienced, and struggled along personal journeys as individuals, while also being pulled in different directions by the group dynamics. As a facilitator there was a constant tension between working for the group to help them to realize their goals, and reasserting control when risks became too high to take. It was not empowerment at its best, partly due to the statutory basis of the project within which the parents' committee operated, and partly because of the tensions inherent in supporting people as they develop within an environment that is new and exciting, but fraught with pitfalls. When I think of empowerment, I think of this group, who as individuals became empowered to various degrees, as a result of the environment creating opportunities for making choices and taking control.

In terms of therapeutic practice, how are these issues relevant? If empowerment is about people being facilitated to take control, make choices and exercise the power they have, and emancipation is about revealing power relations and using this exposure to work towards social change and liberation, what impact do these two concepts have upon practice?

For me, the context I was working in was restrictive. It was a high-profile project and the local media would have relished any uncalculated action

Reflections

Discuss the following questions with a colleague who you can trust.
In what ways is empowerment relevant to your clients?
In what ways is emancipation relevant to your clients?
What are the barriers to incorporating these into practice?

whether on behalf of parent or professional. This did not create a safe space within which to encourage risk-taking and ownership within the parents' group, and created the need for the facilitators to retain some decision-making power within the group. Furthermore, it was a project funded by central government and, therefore, couched within the oppressive social structures that relegated local families to the status of 'disadvantaged'. This created an unequal power relationship immediately, and this was constructed within the project itself. It was, therefore, difficult to take the extra step towards an emancipative approach. Similarly, attitudes were very powerful in shaping the extent to which empowerment was valued. Trust between parents and professionals was a big issue, which in our project was played out around the issue of parental access to the door security code. Additionally retaining the power to define 'these people' and to decide how much power they could handle, was crucial to some professionals, taking on a paternalistic approach of protecting them from themselves. Thus, the shift to an approach of rights and advocacy did not happen on a broader level within the project. The work within the parents' committee was sailing against the tide.

REDUCTIONIST AND DETERMINISTIC VIEWPOINTS

We constantly use stories to understand the world, and to describe our world to other people. Stories are constructions of reality. There are many versions of the same story without one ever being able to be described as the 'truth'. For instance, I may tell the story of my grandparents' deaths to more fully understand my feeling about it each time I tell it. Reality is constructed through the stories we both tell and hear, rather than the stories coldly telling of an already given fact. The events of my grandparents' deaths exist differently for the different people involved because of the different stories each will tell and hear, and the associated stories they know, for instance about family, bereavement, attachment and so on. These associated stories are collected through life, from one's culture, traditions, religion, etc. These may be stories personal to the individual or socially shared narratives. The available stories/narratives about death, e.g. religious, political, moral, etc., the interweaving of all these and my response to them, contribute to my understanding and construction of the meanings of those deaths for me. The stories therapists use to understand reality contribute to what they bring to an encounter with a client. A therapist's stories and understanding about a set of circumstances may differ widely from those of a client, yet somehow these must be negotiated within a therapeutic intervention.

Despite reality being constructed through narratives, some stories exist that are widespread and influence socially shared understandings of reality. Our understanding will be shaped by cultural narratives and our reactions to them, and some of these may be so familiar to us as to be barely perceptible. These narratives are pervasive and can enter consciousness with the force of 'common sense' or other normalizing structures, which make them appear as given and, therefore, not open to question. In terms of working with clients, this can impact upon the starting point, making only certain possibilities tenable.

There are also bigger narratives, such as constructs of 'disability' and 'race', which impose grand generalizations across diverse populations of people across time and space. The perspective known as social constructionism posits that categories of social classification, such as gender, race and disability, are socially constructed rather than innate features of the individual. Such grand narratives reduce diverse peoples down to limiting stereotypes, and impose generalized theories upon them to explain their behaviour. These grand narratives are ideological in that they function to limit and control individuals in society by imposing social norms that people can be measured against as either conforming to or deviating from. These norms create a hierarchy in which those who conform to the most norms come out on top, with a sliding scale down. The norm in the UK is to be white, British, male, young, straight, non-disabled. To deviate is to be classed as 'other'. The more one deviates from this norm, the less power and privilege one is accorded, which translates into social inclusion and participation as a full citizen with all the rights this should grant. Grand narratives sustain this hierarchy and division, by quantifying and labelling the 'differences' that separate people. This creates unequal power relations that then lead to oppression. Empowerment is about individuals resisting this oppression, while emancipation involves revealing the underlying power structures that produce it, and seeking social change to liberate oppressed groups.

In terms of disability, one of the current debates within the disabled people's movement has been around these issues and, in particular, the social model's emphasis on structural barriers, which some have argued has prevented debate about the challenges that an impaired body creates for an individual (Tierney 2002, Crow 1996, Paterson & Hughes 1999). These theorists argue that disability is a complex, multi-layered picture, that cannot be explained by institutional or physical barriers alone. Molloy and Vasil write:

> . . . the split is viewed as problematic because it ignores or denigrates the lived experience of the body and consigns impairment to the domain of medical discourse and authority . . . The second wave writers refocus attention onto impairment in an attempt to redress the abandonment of the body that is the legacy of the social model . . . this turn is part of a

re-socialisation of impairment that allows for accounts of both the lived
experience of impairment and the ways that impairment is discursively
embodied. (2002, p. 663)

The role of the body as a pre-condition for disability oppression, and the
awareness of the physical self created by structural barriers are argued to be
key aspects of disabled people's experience. This debate offers a point of
entry into the arena of the medical versus social model of disability, particularly for therapists whose work with clients may traditionally have been
defined by functional limitation. Beginning to consider issues of the body
within a social model may be a very tangible step in terms of therapists
thinking about empowerment and emancipation within practice.

Grand narratives, such as disability, race and gender, sustain binary
categories. They support the labelling and excluding processes of Western
stratified society, constructing a clear division between the norm and its
opposite, i.e. between black and white, straight and gay, disabled and non-
disabled. This division is portrayed as absolute, with any middle ground
being strongly contested. The opposite is always viewed negatively, while the
notion of the norm is protected from the reality that it only makes sense as a
category in relation to its supposed opposite. helen (charles) writes:

Being white seems to be nice and simple . . . For example, 'whiteness' is
still not being widely seen in this country, northern Europe, or North
America as an ethnicity, as a colour, as pertaining to anything to do with
'race'. Why? . . . I have often wondered whether white people *know* that
they are white . . . And if they do, is it only when their notion of the
'other' as 'non-white' is placed before them? Is it only when the binary
opposition of white and 'black' or 'Asian' is within their field of vision?
And can they only speak for themselves from the borrowed position of
who they construe as 'other'? (1993, p. 99)

In dominant ideology, the existence of groups defined by binary opposites is
not generally questioned. The innate existence of male and female attributes
within men and women, for instance, is widely accepted. What is also not
commonly questioned, except in resistance politics, however, is what led to
social inequality being attached to physical characteristics such as sex, skin
colour and impairment. It was only in the Stephen Lawrence inquiry that
racism was formally recognized as 'institutionalized', i.e. created and sustained through social structures, and not merely a product of individual
prejudice. However, the reality remains that institutional barriers are

maintained for all 'others', yet this is concealed through 'otherness' being inscribed individually through dominant models that are used to tie experience to the individual, such as the medical model of disability. These reductionistic perspectives make those who are institutionally excluded responsible for that exclusion.

As these messages are so pervasive it is unsurprising that many clients are already grounded within this perspective, feeling quite alone and unique in their situation and focusing upon functional limitation. It may be some time before a client is ready to think about the structural and institutional barriers that construct their impairment as disability, and to begin to reformulate their identity within this new framework. Other clients may not see themselves as disabled and never integrate this within their own identity. For other clients, their impairment may fall within the gaps between what is socially constructed as a disability and what is not, causing tensions between their lived experience and the external perceptions of others. This often happens for clients with a hidden disability, or for whom their impairment is contested as a disability at all, for instance obesity and anorexia. These clients offer evidence that the supposed clear divide between the categories of disabled and non-disabled is in fact false.

Those who refuse or fail to conform to binary categorization are often treated with more suspicion than those perceived as the opposite to the norm – for instance, bisexuals, transsexuals, those of mixed racial parentage, lesbians who have been married – and the validity of their identities is often questioned. This leads to the non-articulation of these realities, through the lack of linguistic structures and concepts to describe a reality felt by the wider society to not exist. Mason-John & Khambatta grapple with the term 'mixed race' as a means of representing their diverse cultural heritage against the backdrop of the black–white binary of racial identification:

> The term mixed race, while an improvement on half-caste, is still regarded as an inexact shorthand for being born of one white and one black parent. Not all of us who are racially 'mixed' conform to this model. The term mixed racial parentage has possibilities, but still defines us on the basis of the racial background of our parents, ignoring the fact that for some of us the racial 'mix' occurred further back than this. (1993, p. 36)

These alternative spaces that deny the validity of binary thinking offer opportunities to construct different stories about identity, self and reality, and stories from these spaces can enable us to re-think our own stories and our approach to the world and the way in which we understand it. D'Aoust describes the 'maps' she uses to locate herself across spaces that continually segregate her coexisting identities into more manageable chunks, and the strategies she uses to help others to put all the pieces together and to deal with her as a holistic individual. She also discusses the identities others impose onto her in order to make sense of her without shifting any of their preconceived assumptions. She writes:

Naming these experiences, which are all a part of who I am, short of an autobiography, helps me to present myself to the unknown reader in categories commonly understood (misunderstood?). Nonetheless, I am still me.

The map is not the territory, the name is not the thing, my (your) labels are not me . . .

. . . In many cultures, the concept of naming has deceived people into thinking the map (which is the representation of the thing) is the territory (the thing) . . . I am not what people label me to be. I am me . . .

. . . My opinion on maps is that their importance to others has a significant impact on my life and the lives of others who are mapped . . .

. . . I can only try to be clear about what I map internally, and what I project externally. I know that by using my own maps and naming these maps to the outside world that people who meet me will accept and maybe understand my territories and how they are mapped by language. (1996, pp. 154, 155, 163)

The concept of maps is akin to my use of the term stories/narratives. These are crucial in the way therapists perceive and respond to clients, and the foundations upon which an enabling relationship can be built.

The following theories of feminism, symbolic interactionism and existential psychology will offer ways of making these ideas concrete within practice, and suggest ways of trying out new narratives by which to construct the relationship between yourself and your client.

FEMINISM

Feminism broadly represents a system of thought that makes the overarching narrative of gender apparent, rejecting it as a 'truth'. Gender is, rather, constructed as a power relationship designed to stratify society into two groups, giving one considerably more power and privilege, assigning roles and relationships, and creating expectations, assumptions and norms to be adhered to. The critique of gender as a power relationship specifically focuses on women's inferior social position in relation to men and seeks the empowerment and emancipation of women as an oppressed group. Feminism is a broad philosophy and within it theorists influenced by a diversity of other schools of thought create its theories. Thus, feminism is not a single, consistent philosophy and political movement, but a discursive site within which a range of perspectives compete for dominance. One strand of this competition is between a modern and postmodern view of feminism, and the politics that would achieve its aims. Modern feminism seeks to re-value the female at the expense of the male to create equality, while postmodern feminism champions the deconstruction of the system upon which the artificial division of gender is based, thus ending the necessity for the male/female distinction. This involves paying attention more to the workings of power and its deployment in order to identify ways of intervening in this.

In addition to this debate about what feminism is and what politics best suit its agenda, feminist writers also grapple with the interplay with gender of other axes of social stratification, such as race, sexuality, disability, age and religion. Martin wrote:

> . . . differences, for example, of race, class or sexuality, are finally rendered noncontradictory by virtue of their (re)presentation as differences between individuals, reducible to questions of identity within the unifying context of feminism. What remains unexamined are the systematic institutional relationships between those differences, relationships that exceed the boundaries of the lesbian community, the women's movement, or particular individuals, and in which apparently bounded communities and individuals are deeply implicated. (1988, p. 78)

This links, interestingly, to the debate between the medical and social model of disability, as a criticism of the medical model is that it ties disability to the individual, leaving unexamined the systematic institutional relationships that turn impairment into disability. For me, the most powerful feminist writers are those who recognize the interrelationship of different axes of social stratification – for instance, those who acknowledge that race will impact upon the experience of gender, while disability will impact upon sexuality, and so on and so forth. This both acknowledges the crucial differences between women as a diverse group, and locates the construction of the social meaning of those differences within institutional structures of stratification. Taking a wide view of oppression and power relationships I believe enhances theorizing around a single issue such as gender. Thus, theorists within political movements that challenge oppression through race, disability, age, etc., have much to offer feminism, and vice versa, in terms of understanding reductionist thinking and its impact upon oppression and empowerment.

Gender itself is a social construct that separates the sexes and imposes norms of appearance and behaviour upon them. From this, assumptions, stereotypes and identities are created, from which it is socially discouraged to deviate. A famously coined feminist phrase is that 'the personal is political'. This means that all those elements of a personal life that traditionally were seen as private, and as unworthy of attention are actually crucial in understanding the operation of power within the system of gender (and other axes of social stratification). A feminist approach considers the impact of gender as the key to understanding all other aspects of a life, by illuminating the nature and impact of the gendered social world. This is directly relevant to working within enabling relationships, as everything each gendered being does has a social significance that is both shaped and determined by, and simultaneously helps to shape and determine, gender. For instance, the norms around body image and the social value attached to women as a result of appearance may figure highly if the problem presented impacts upon this. A young woman with Down's syndrome may experience low self-esteem as all the visual images in our culture silently communicate to her that she is unacceptable, and unvaluable within the economy of beauty that is traded through the media.

The diagnosis a person receives will become meaningful in relation to social narratives such as gender, when one considers what kind of lives society expect men and women to have, and what is socially sanctioned. For instance, a young man with a muscle-wasting condition will feel the impact of the stereotypes around masculinity and manhood, and his growing inability to live up to these. The imperative to conform is powerful, and yet basing one's intervention on working to enable clients to come more into line with the socially sanctioned images of acceptable gender will not solve the problem and only perpetuates the person's oppression. If it is the client's goal to conform, however, then the therapist will need to think carefully about the ways other choices and options could be presented, without disempowering the client by labelling their original goal as invalid.

Reflections

Discuss the following questions with a colleague who you can trust.
What are your own values and beliefs in relation to cultural norms and the impetus to conform to them?
What are the implications of setting therapeutic goals that perpetuate the aim of making up for the implied deficit of the client?

The client's relationships with the therapist and with others, feminists would argue, are mediated by gender through socially agreed roles, behaviours, and expectations and the meanings attached to actions performed by each gender. The relationships available between individuals within such confines can be as restrictive as the identities available, unless, again, alternatives are created and negotiated. Power relations are criticized within feminism as being inherently abusive, and yet a power relationship exists between therapist and client, which will be complexly mediated by other social structures that will position each person in relation to the other. The therapist is in a position of power as the 'expert' on the particular problem the client is experiencing, and, therefore, has the power to label the client with a diagnosis, and to base this diagnosis on maps that the client may not use to define their own territory. Negotiating an equal relationship within such a situation may be impossible.

Reflections

Consider what forms of power come with being a therapist.
In what ways has this been mediated in your experience of working with clients?
What steps can you take to build a more empowering relationship with clients, and what might be the barriers to this?

Rather than seeking to create equality within a relationship where this may be socially impossible, a therapist can attempt to work to create an 'anti-oppressive' relationship. This acknowledges power differentials, but seeks to minimize their impact within the relationship, by making them explicit and actively working to prevent the oppressive use of power within the relationship. This would involve both acknowledging the ways in which therapist and client were positioned in relation to each other in a wider social context, and avoiding the erasure or denial of experiences that appear to fall outside the remit of the therapeutic relationship. For instance, that the client is a lesbian may appear irrelevant to the therapy, yet it will impact upon the other identities that a diagnosis of their difficulties might bring, and will figure in the client's understanding of, and response to, the diagnosis and intervention. This involves having wide parameters of possibility that people can be and become, as if our personal narrative boundaries prevent us, for instance, seeing disabled mothers as lesbian women. Professionals can limit who clients can be within therapy practice. Creating therapeutic solutions *with* clients involves interaction and dialogue. Marks writes:

> . . . the process of learning is centred around the client who requires space and time in order to explore their own position and experience within the world. Change emerges out of a collaboration between client and professional. (2002, p. 3)

It involves renegotiating power and control of the therapy, being non-judgemental, recognizing the unequal social structures created by race, gender, age, etc., and being committed to not replicating these within the therapeutic relationship.

SYMBOLIC INTERACTION

Symbolic interaction refers to a sociological and social psychological approach to understanding human interaction and group dynamics, where reality is believed to be constructed through the interactions that occur between people, rather than reality being a pre-existent entity. Blumer's theory (1989) is recognized as a basis of the approach, and this is founded upon several assumptions. The way we act towards things is based upon the meaning they have for us, while these meanings arise out of social interactions. Tierney writes:

> The type of impairment someone has, and the way it is socially constructed, influences how others treat and interrelate with her/him. (2002, p. 9)

The social meaning of impairment will significantly impact upon the meaning a diagnosis will have for a client, and the attitudes towards impairment, and themselves as an impaired person will be influential in the way the client continues to deal with the problem. Crisp suggests that the way clients understand their impairment will be reflected in the language that they use to describe it. He writes:

> Rehabilitation counsellors should therefore conceptualise disability via the exploration of the meanings behind the language used by persons with disabilities instead of accepting common understandings or generalisations of disability. (2002, p. 23)

Thus, part of the role of the therapist may be to intervene in the construction of meaning around the impairment, to work with the client to construct meanings that are more empowering. Working explicitly from the social model of disability involves helping the client to identify the social barriers that construct the impairment as a disability.

As the meanings we attach to ourselves, others, our environment, objects and relationships will be constructed through interpersonal interactions, these meanings will be negotiated and renegotiated over time, making meaning unstable and ever changing. This creates the possibility for the therapist to intervene in the process of meaning construction for the client, and to work towards empowering interpretations. The availability of a range of perspectives, with none being able to be defined as the 'truth' opens up the space to consider other ways of thinking about impairment. Crisp writes:

> ... clients are encouraged: to see themselves in relation to a problem instead of having, or being, a problem; to value multiple points of view; to view self as being defined by a diversity of experiential contexts; and to expand their conceptualisations concerning the link between self and society. (2002, p. 24)

This is a key concept for therapists, as the meaning of the client's problem will be constantly renegotiated within the therapeutic relationship. Conversely, however, the therapist also has the potential to reinforce oppressive meanings around impairment and create disabling barriers for clients through the perpetuation of dominant stereotypes.

According to Blumer (1989), meanings are adapted within interactions through a process of interpretation and self-reflection. We take away new experiences from a social encounter, and then reflect upon their implication for ourselves. Each session with the therapist will feature for clients as a key social encounter, from which they will take away experiences that they will later reflect upon, and use to continuously reconstruct their own understanding. The models offered to clients by therapists to understand their difficulties will strongly impact upon the client's personal concept of themselves (their narrative, map, identity, etc.). This is the opportunity for the therapist and client to work together, using the contact time as a social encounter within which new, shared meanings can be created.

Finally, Blumer asserts that the meanings things have for an individual are shaped by a complex process of interpretation that is linked to the production and consumption of cultural texts (images, objects, fiction, etc.) within society. Thus, the products of mass media profoundly impact upon the meaning things have for us. This impact extends to the meanings that identities have for us, such as those that are shaped by gender, race, ability, age, etc. Lindesmith states:

These identities are attached to representations of family, race, age, gender, nationality, and social class. These objects and identities are in turn located in an ongoing political economy, which is a complex, interconnected system. The political economy structures the *production*, *distribution*, and *consumption* of wealth in a society. It determines the 'who, what, when, where, why, and how' of wealth and power in every-day life – that is, who gets what income, at what time, in what places, for what labour, and why. This economy *regulates* the production, distribution, and consumption of cultural objects. It does so by repeatedly forming links that connect cultural objects (cars, clothing, food, houses), their material representations, and the personal identities of consumers as gendered human beings. (1999, p. 12)

The impact of media on our constructions of selves and others, and identities can be profound and can lock us into ways of interacting that perpetuate the status quo and reinforce identities that individuals may not choose for themselves. The display of images, in health care centres, that challenge stereo-typical identities can introduce alternative narratives about impairment. It is also important for therapists to be aware of the ways in which media products will impact upon the construction of their own meanings, around the work they do and the clients' difficulties. Becoming more aware and critical of this is a similar process to coming to understand gender as a social construct from a feminist perspective.

EXISTENTIAL PSYCHOLOGY

Existential psychology comes under a humanist approach that developed in opposition to behaviourist and psychoanalytical approaches to mental health. The behaviourist approach conceptualized mental health as the absence of pathological symptoms, while psychoanalysis defined it as maintaining the balance between unconscious desires and the constraints of reality. Both work from a deficit model. In contrast, humanistic psychology defined mental health as psychological growth and development, with Carl Rogers (1902–1987) defining self-actualization as a key factor within this. Existentialist theory argues that people are always responsible for their actions, and that they have free will and the right to choose. The data then with which to study humans are defined as the choices they make. This is phenomenolog-ical in many ways, as the study of experience is viewed as more important than the study of behaviour. RD Laing was a key exponent of existential psychology, and he challenged existing perceptions of mental health, by describing schizo-phrenia as a choice to retreat from reality, rather than something that affected a client and which they had no control over. This, Laing argued, re-empowered the client, and took them out of the clutches of a powerful condition that pre-viously they had been defined as being at the mercy of. It also ran the risk of 'blaming' the client, however, as people could then believe the client had the will to choose to 'snap out of it'. Thus, Laing argued that understanding the objective reality of the patient was not important. What was important, he claimed, was to understand the person's experience of their reality, and to understand how she/he viewed the problem (Hayes 2000).

From this viewpoint, therapy practice involves understanding the problem from the client's perspective, and therapists using their expertise to work with the client to find solutions. This is a collaborative approach and requires partnership, which involves empowerment in terms of choice and decision-making and, more importantly, in terms of whose interpretation of the situation is given prominence. This can also work conversely, in that therapists can help to change the way clients view the problem, to move them from thinking purely about functional limitation, and onto the social barriers created for them and how these could be removed and challenged.

Laing went on to argue that giving a diagnosis was not an objective act, but instead involved applying social judgements and attaching a label. The social judgement is that the person deviates sufficiently from the 'norm', while the label characterizes the nature of the deviance and signifies an appropriate social response. Furthermore, giving a diagnosis involves the person applying the label taking charge, being in control and having the power, which in turn leads to the client losing all these things. Thompson (1993) argues that a clinical diagnosis leads to an incomplete and obstructive view of the individual, as it takes a single strand of a complex whole, and presents this as the defining piece of the complex picture. The label can then come to define the person, rather than merely being seen as a single feature of their experience. For example, in medical terminology people may be described as their conditions, such as being 'a right hemiplegia', 'a spina bifida', or 'the muscular dystrophy boys'. These labels describe how she/he should be perceived and treated by others and legitimate the continued oppression of marginalized groups of people. Laing argued that schizophrenia was a label imposed from outside as a means of preserving the status quo, and relegating any alternative perceptions of society to the realms of 'madness'. He argued people labelled as schizophrenics were society's greatest critics (Gross 2001).

Laing went on to argue that the concept of mental health is constructed in the interactions between people, rather than residing within an individual. Thus, again, mental ill health is not an innate feature located within an individual, but a social interpretation based upon perceived norms of social interaction. He also argued that the conventional borders of the binary division between mental health and mental ill health were not as clearly defined as thought, and that this was a matter of perception and interpretation rather

Reflections

Discuss the following questions with a colleague who you can trust.
In what ways can a diagnosis or label for a client's difficulties help or hinder your intervention with a client?
What are the implications for empowering and/or emancipatory practice?

than of clearly definable categories. The label of mental ill health could be used to outlaw 'anti-social' acts, such as young unmarried pregnancy, homosexuality, criminality, etc., and it was used as such well into the 1900s. This is linked to the meanings attached to things, how reality is perceived and how perceiving is normalized through the creation of an outlawed mode of perception. It is the social interpretation of the behaviour that constructs it as an impairment, rather than anything inherently within the behaviour itself. This is illustrated in the case of Asperger syndrome. Molloy & Vasil question how this diagnostic category of Asperger syndrome has been constructed and in whose interests. They highlight the range of factors that contribute to a diagnosis being made stating:

> The common rhetoric of the child's needs conflates a range of different needs: the need of the school to maintain order and to function smoothly; the needs of the parents to make sense of their child's behaviour; the needs of the speech therapist and occupational therapist to have a common methodology and concomitant professional language to support their practice. (2002, p. 666)

Understanding how the client views the world/problem and developing an empowering understanding is key to working towards a solution. This involves giving up the mantle of the expert, and instead allowing the client to define his/her own reality and lead the therapist towards the right conclusion (Gross 2001).

Carl Rogers, a key humanist psychologist, argued that the quality of the enabling relationship set the ground for the client in solving his/her own problem, as it was the therapist's job to create a safe and accepting space, within which the client had the confidence to grow and self-actualize. Rogers argued that the person best placed to solve a client's problems was the client, but what she/he needed, and prior to therapy had lacked, was a safe space within which to grow. The client's perceptions of his/her mobility, environmental or speech problem will give key clues to the best approach to solving the problem (Hayes 2000). Treating the problem as the client sees it is the key to existential psychology. It also links to an empowering approach as the transferring of the role of the expert from therapist to client can begin a process of choice and decision-making.

CONCLUSION

The three perspectives outlined above have many overlapping features. Both existential psychology and symbolic interactionism place a great deal of emphasis on the meanings attached to things, and the construction of these meanings through social encounters. Feminism too looks at meanings in terms of the ways gender mediates interpretation. For both existential psychology and symbolic interactionism, relationships are key to the construction of reality, to the formulation of problems, and to the social significance these will have. Within feminism, relationships are characterized by power relations that must be negotiated in order for empowerment to occur. For all three perspectives, the ability to step back from the dominant social narratives and re-evaluate what might be going on for clients in terms of the way they have been labelled, the meanings attached to their diagnosis, and the stereotypes associated with their identities, is clearly central to the philosophy. Furthermore, the message from all three is that if the therapy is not part of the solution, then it is part of the problem, and actively contributing to disempowering social relations.

Chapter 6

From theory to principles
John Swain

This chapter attempts to provide a bridge between context (professional structures, ethics and values, understandings of human relations, theory) and therapy practice. In terms of the structure of the book it is also a bridge between Parts 1 and 2 ('In context' and 'In theory and principle') and Part 3 ('In practice'). The search for principles to guide practice is certainly not a new endeavour.

To set the scene for the framework of principles developed here, I shall briefly outline two existing examples of what can be broadly called 'critical' approaches. Thompson (1998, 2001) has developed a PCS analysis in understanding inequalities and discrimination experienced by clients, as a foundation for bridging theory and practice. There are three levels of analysis that are closely interlinked and interact with each other. The P level is the *personal* or *psychological*; it incorporates the individual's thoughts, feelings and attitudes, including prejudice and actions. This level also includes practice in the sense of the analysis of interactions between practitioner and client. The C level is the *cultural*, incorporating shared ways of seeing, thinking and doing – shared meanings. S refers to the *structural* level that generally includes power relations and structures, and incorporates institutional discrimination and processes of social change towards equality and justice. This analysis can underpin a range of strategies to promote equality by challenging discrimination and oppression. Thompson states: 'Empowerment, by assisting people to take greater control over their lives, can have a significant positive impact at the personal level, thereby making a contribution at the cultural level and, in turn, playing at least a small part in undermining inequality at the

Reflections

Principles are ideals towards which therapy practice is directed and against which practice is reflected on. What principles do you adhere to? You may find it useful at this point to stop and think, discuss with colleagues and jot down a few notes about the principles that underpin your practice.

structural level' (1998, p. 212). From this broad basis, reflective practice enables practitioners to take account of a range of factors at the personal, cultural and structural levels.

In the volume edited by Brechin et al. critical reflection is incorporated into a broader idea of critical practice:

> The term 'critical' is used here to refer to open-minded, reflective appraisal that takes account of different perspectives, experiences and assumptions. (2000, p. 26)

As with Thompson, processes of empowerment and anti-oppression are seen as crucial. She picks out two overall guiding principles. The first is the principle of 'respecting others as equals' (2000, p. 31). This is justified, in part, by the 'endemic oppression of less powerful groups in society' (2000, p. 31). The second guiding principle is openness. This is an acceptance of the position that there is a degree of uncertainty in all professional practice and that professional practice is evolving within the particular social and historical context. Dewey defined openness as follows:

> Active desire to listen to more sides than one, to give heed to facts from whatever source they come, to give full attention to alternative possibilities, to recognise the possibility of error even in the beliefs that are dearest to us. (1933, p. 29)

Founded on these principles, Brechin et al. go on to outline three pillars of critical practice: forging relationships, seeking to empower others and making a difference.

The framework of principles developed in this chapter shares many of the elements of the two approaches described above. This framework is depicted in Figure 6.1. It encompasses three arenas for relating theory to practice: enabling relationships, processes of critical reflection, and empowerment and emancipation. It offers a map for questioning practice derived from theory. As such it must be viewed within a number of imperatives. What sort of map is this?

1. The arenas are closely interlinked and interact with each other. It is not possible to consider questions of enabling relationships as distinct from principles of critical reflection or empowerment and emancipation.
2. All the concepts within this framework have multiple meanings. This model is built on nebulous concepts: participation, partnership, reflection, empowerment and emancipation. These are concepts with multiple meanings, depending on who is using them, in what contexts and for what purposes. These are ideals or values that must themselves be continuously the focus of critical reflection.
3. It is one possible framework. It is a sounding board of ideas against which you can address your own beliefs, views and feelings.

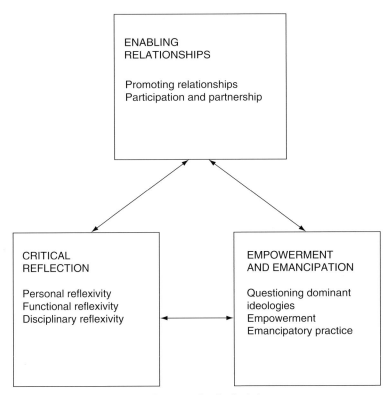

Fig. 6.1   An enabling relationships framework of principles

CRITICAL REFLECTION

Critical reflection is included as integral to the framework of principles on the basis that good practice should be critically reflective practice. Gould writes of the value of reflective practice:

> There is considerable empirical evidence, based on research into a variety of occupations, suggesting that expertise does not derive from the application of rules or procedures applied deductively from positivist research. Instead, it is argued that practice wisdom rests upon highly developed intuition which can be difficult to articulate but can be demonstrated in practice. (1996, p. 1)

The idea of reflective practice is, in part, based on the notion that uncertainty is built into all therapy practice and, indeed, professional practice. This is clear, for instance, when considering ethics: dilemmas pervade the whole therapy process and can be generated by differing rights, responsibilities, motivations, aspirations and vested interests of all concerned. The processes of ethical decision-making need themselves to be subjected to critical analysis by all concerned (see Chapter 3). Flexibility is essential in broaching uncertainty and the unique situations faced daily by therapists (Thompson 2000). Central to the origins of the notion of reflective practice is an understanding of professional knowledge as developed by practitioners themselves through and within their practice and their systematic analysis of practice.

These ideas have been developed in different ways and in a variety of contexts. Ghaye and his colleagues have produced a series of books on reflection for health-care professionals. Ghaye & Lillyman (2000, p. 121) offer a framework of twelve principles of reflection with particular emphasis on the first three:

1. Reflective practice is about you and your work.
2. Reflective practice is about learning from experience.
3. Reflective practice is about valuing what we do and why we do it.

The 'father' of these developments is generally acknowledged to be Donald Schön (1983, 1987). His work has been widely adopted, and adapted, in professional training and development. He distinguishes between two models of theories-in-use or theories-in-action. Model I, sometimes referred to as the traditional model, involves the following action strategies for the therapist: design and managing the environment so that the therapist is in control of the factors that he or she sees as relevant; own and control the task; unilaterally protect him/herself by, for instance, withholding critical information; and unilaterally protect others, particularly the client, from being hurt. Schön associated this model with what he calls 'single loop' learning: 'Learning about strategies or tactics for achieving one's own objectives' (1987, p. 256). Model II, or the reflective practice model, is characterized by quite different action strategies including: design situations in which the participants, particularly the therapist and client, are involved in defining and controlling relevant factors; the task is jointly controlled; and protection of self and others is a joint enterprise and orientated towards mutual growth.

A crucial dimension of model II is the wider social and historical, albeit professional, context. The ripples of understanding move outwards in ever increasing circles. For instance, to reflect on the therapist–client relationship in the context of the professional role of the therapist raises a whole series of questions about being a therapist:

1. How does each therapist adopt and adapt to a professional role? What implications and meaning does this have for how therapists relate to clients?
2. How does any particular body of professionals define the professional role? What requirements, for instance, does a speech and language therapist have to fulfil in providing speech and language therapy?
3. Why and how has a particular body of professionals been established at this particular time and in this particular form? Why has a particular arena of expertise, such as knowledge and skills in speech and language therapy, been recognized as the domain and exclusive territory of one specific group of professionals?

Reflections

Schön writes:

> Practitioners do reflect on their knowledge-in-practice. Sometimes in the relative tranquillity of a post-mortem, they think back on a project they have undertaken, a situation they have lived through, and they explore the understandings they have brought to their handling of the case. (1983, p. 61)

There are a number of possible modes of reflection including: conversations in the head, informal conversations, written records, discussions with a colleague who can act as a critical friend, and more formal arrangements for supervision or appraisal. One common form of retrospective reflection is writing a journal. You will find some guidelines in the Introduction. Some practitioners, sometimes to their surprise, have found this to be a powerful process. As Ghaye & Lillyman point out, there are risks as well as benefits associated with journal writing. There are a number of ethical issues to be resolved and a code of practice to be established. They state:

> For example, there is the issue of 'rights'. Who has the right to decide what is written and shared? Is it wise to assume that we have the right to keep what is written private and confidential? (2000, pp. 106–107)

For those who do not develop and clarify their thinking by writing, journal writing can be little more than a chore. The first thing to say, then, is that though it can be worth persevering, if writing a journal is not a good mode of reflection for you, then simply put it aside and concentrate on other ways of reflecting. Furthermore, it is important not to think of keeping a journal as something that you might or might not be doing correctly. There is no set formula for writing a journal. If it is a good mode of reflection for you, you will find your own style, content and even audience. On the last of these, for instance, one student wrote as if to another person. She addressed her journal to a pretend critical friend and found this the most effective for her. You should develop your own approach to keeping a journal.

Despite the prevalence of the reflective practice approach, there are certain problems. There is a presumption in the approach that the practitioner has unproblematic access to their biases, feelings, motivations and so on. Self-awareness is tenuous and nebulous. As Gough & McFadden point out, the task becomes even more onerous with a post-modern view of self:

> How can you pin down a self which is multi-faceted, dynamic and embedded in language and social relationships? (2001, p. 68)

Furthermore, reflection does invoke a broader context, but it tends to be the professional context. Schön makes little or no reference to the broader social and historical context. Thompson (2000) points out that the significance of gender, culture, disability and so on is essentially peripheral. The need for critical reflection calls for a broader framework of analysis. It is in this light that we turn to the enabling relationships framework of principles, as depicted in Figure 6.1.

First, critical reflection is integral to the framework alongside and closely interconnected with both social relationships and issues of power in social relations. Three distinct forms of reflexivity are recognized drawing on Wilkinson's (1988) work: personal, functional and disciplinary. The notion of critical reflection is certainly not confined to the reflective practice approach. Reflexivity, albeit in different guises, has played a broad role in the social sciences. Indeed, Giddens argues that what he calls the 'late modern' age of Western society is a time of high reflexivity. He defines 'self-identity' as 'the self reflexively understood by the person in terms of her or his biography' (1991, p. 53). One significant arena for the development of reflexivity has been qualitative research where it is perhaps the most distinctive feature (Banister et al. 1994). Wilkinson's model of reflexivity comes from research from a feminist perspective, in which a participative and open stance is advocated.

Personal reflexivity

This is about acknowledging who you are, how your personal interests and values contribute to the construction of the therapy process from initiation to completion – and also being explicit about this. As pointed out above such self-awareness is clearly important in principle, but is highly problematic in practice. It depends, in the first instance, on an understanding of what 'self' is. Thompson (2000, p. 117), drawing on the work of Gambrill (1990), argues that by recognizing the person as a central feature of human resource development, we also recognize the key role of self-awareness. This applies to your strengths, weaknesses and characteristic patterns in relation to: knowledge – with the recognition that facts do not speak for themselves and knowledge is through interpretation and giving meaning; skills – with the recognition that these are 'people skills' not 'mechanical skills' and part of interpersonal/ relationship dynamics; and values – which are cultural as well as personal. This is, in slightly different guises, quite a common model for understanding human beings in various contexts. Attitudes, for instance, are commonly broken down into ideas/knowledge, behaviour/actions and emotions/ feelings.

The notion of self-awareness becomes questionable, from the perspective of enabling relationships, in that it can be individualistic and removed from the context of personal relationships and culture. There is no recognition, then, that self-awareness is a cultural imperative in present-day Western society, as evidenced, for instance, with the growth of psychotherapeutic and counselling services. Yet, clearly, we need to develop a reflexive quality, to be critically analytic at a number of levels and know ourselves within the broader context of personal relationships and social relations, as a foundation for developing enabling relationships.

The notion of 'values' has been extensively used in empowering and anti-oppressive practice (Braye & Preston-Shoot 1995, Dalrymple & Burke 1995). Values are sets of beliefs, ideas and assumptions, infused with personal feelings. They weave and interweave different levels. On a collective basis they provide form and meaning to culture – and also differentiate between cultures. At an interpersonal level, they define and influence how we think and act between us. There is also a professional level, with values inherent in professional organizations, procedures, responsibilities and so on. Values are essentially shared, but they are also essentially competing and conflicting both within and between levels. Enabling relationships, then, is founded, in part, on critical reflection, analysis and action on principles that are collectively valued and embedded in society's structure and constructed in interpersonal communication and relationships.

Braye & Preston-Shoot (1995) distinguish between 'traditional' and 'radical' values, echoing recurring themes in earlier chapters in this book. Traditional values can be associated with a reformist agenda based on key assumptions that:

- inequalities are inevitable given the natural differences there are between people
- inequalities are an inevitable feature of social organization
- a caring society will provide for those unable through incapacity and disadvantage to improve their own lot
- individuals, given equal opportunity, have the potential to remove barriers to personal success and are themselves responsible for doing so.

Radical values can be associated with the need for structural change based on key assumptions that:

- an individual's life chances are determined by her or his position in society's structure
- society's structure is best understood in terms of social divisions that differentiate between groups of people
- inequalities exist in the relative power held by such groups to gain and sustain valued resources and advantages
- the care and services provided by society can justify and support inequalities
- individual need is part of a collective experience shared by a group of people
- inequality and social change must be addressed through collective action.

Finally, personal reflection is not necessarily a focus on the individual, nor is it necessarily an individual activity. Returning to reflection in qualitative research, for many this is pursued through participative and co-operative strategies. Hollway, for instance, found that a variety of activities increased her 'understanding of self and others': 'writing a journal, recording my dreams, being a member of women's consciousness raising groups, teaching group dynamics through experiential methods and above all, talking end-lessly to friends – about them and about me' (1989, p. 2).

Functional reflexivity

With slight re-wording, Wilkinson (1988, p. 495) defines this as entailing: continuous critical examination of the practice/process of therapy to reveal its assumptions, values and biases. In a research study of therapy (in particular occupational therapy), Barnitt argued that therapists struggle with the tension of doing good to the client and doing good to themselves as therapists in a profession with professional expectations and hierarchical power relations: 'Therapists were not free to make independent, personally virtuous decisions, as on many occasions they had to take into account other participants' wishes, in particular those of people who were more senior in the health hierarchy and patients, relatives and carers who claim increasing rights over services' (2000, p. 110). This, however, does not recognize that therapists may make independent, personally virtuous decisions to take into account other participants' wishes. The key issue within functional reflexivity is the distribution of power and status within therapy.

Disciplinary reflexivity

Disciplinary reflexivity involves a critical stance towards therapy within broader debates about theory and practice. Thompson (2000) argues the significance of theory for practice on a number of grounds. First, theory contributes to the development of anti-discriminatory practice: 'Indeed, theory has a very important role to play in this respect in terms of its capacity for "debunking" (2000, p. 31). Basically, theory is needed to develop a critical perspective to interrogate the values, interactions and context that have shaped and defined therapy practice. Second, practice is inextricably bound to theory, whether formal, 'book' theory, or informal. Fish & Coles (2000) contrast two views of professional practice in analyzing the relationship between theory and practice. The technical rational view of professionalism sees practice as a basic matter of delivering services to clients through a predetermined set of clear-cut routines and behaviours. In the professional artistry view, practice involves in-built uncertainty requiring complex decisions relying on a mixture of judgement, intuition and common sense. A professional artistry view that challenges dogma in therapy practice seems to me to be compatible with the enabling relationships framework.

The following three general principles complete this section on critical reflection:

- To promote understanding of self and others through personal reflection and through dialogue.
- To facilitate functional reflection through critical examination of the practice/process of therapy to reveal its assumptions, values and biases.
- To develop disciplinary reflection and a critical stance towards therapy within broader debates about theory and practice.

ENABLING RELATIONSHIPS

Promoting relationships

For Brechin (2000) the first pillar of becoming a critical practitioner is forging relationships with people, whether clients or colleagues. Therapy practice is constructed from start to finish through interpersonal relationships that are themselves constituted through communication. Forging 'good' relationships and building communication is, of course, central. This includes diverse, challenging and fundamentally uncertain and problematic circumstances. It involves flexibility in establishing dialogue, negotiating, mediating and challenging. As Brechin (2000, p. 36) recognizes, this will involve multiple roles and a range of relationships: professional–client, professional–team, interorganizational, purchaser–provider, supervisor–learner, manager–staff, relationships with policy-makers or politicians, and relationships with the media or the public.

Participation and partnership

The terms 'participation' and 'partnership' are used here to denote the inclusion of clients' voices in decision-making in therapy practice. This is the principle of working with rather than on people. A partnership approach involves participation in decision-making in the therapy process (Thompson 1998, p. 213): identifying problems to be tackled, issues to be addressed and goals to be achieved; deciding what steps are to be taken and who needs to do what; undertaking the necessary work through collaboration and consultation; reviewing progress and agreeing any changes that need to be made to the agreed course of action; bringing the work to a close if and when necessary; and evaluating the work done, highlighting strengths, weaknesses and lessons to be learned.

In recent policy developments, partnership has been a dominant concept signifying the attainment of greater equality in professional–client relations generally. Defining the concept of partnership, however, is difficult because partnership means different things to different groups of people. Broadly, it refers to organizations or individuals working together or acting jointly. Partnership can also be represented as a core principle or an attitudinal stance, based on a fundamental shift of power (Stevenson & Parsloe 1993). Partnerships between professionals and clients are predicated on some expectation of an increase in choice for those receiving services. Any real choice, however, may be a mirage as choice can be seen as a threat by professionals who act as gatekeepers by continuing to make the decisions about access to provision.

The search for principles to guide participation and partnerships is not a new endeavour. Brechin & Swain (1989, p. 51) developed 'six principles of practice' for a 'working alliance' between professionals and people with learning difficulties that attempted to recognize that client involvement must be on the client's terms. From the perspective of people with learning difficulties participation and partnership should be seen as:

1. an entitlement rather than an imposition
2. promoting self-realization rather than compliance
3. opening up choices, rather than replacing one choice with another
4. developing opportunities, relationships and patterns of living in line with their individual wishes, rather than rule-of-thumb normality
5. enhancing their decision-making control of their own lives
6. allowing them to move at their own pace.

As you saw in Chapter 2, there are a number of possible organizational barriers to working in partnership. Beresford et al. (2000, pp. 191–192) points to more psychological barriers. First, clients can themselves be disempowered. People who have spent a considerable period, sometimes a lifetime, without control over the decisions that affect their lives can experience difficulties in participating on an equal basis with professionals perceived as 'the experts'. Helplessness is a psychological state that can result when events and outcomes are uncontrollable – that is, they are independent of a person's responses and behaviour. The psychological consequences of powerlessness are an important dimension of the roles imposed on oppressed groups: 'always a feeling of powerlessness – the feeling that one is black, female, working class, disabled or whatever, things are the way they are and one simply has to accept them because one doesn't have the power to change them' (Sutherland 1981, p. 43). Second, fears and anxieties on both sides can be obstacles to open dialogue. Client participation in decision-making can be threatening to professionals in fulfilling their responsibilities, often in the context of organizational change.

The following two general principles complete this section on enabling relationships:

- To promote mutual understanding and awareness of others' preferences, wishes and needs through open two-way communication.
- To facilitate, through working in partnership, a collaborative approach to service organization, planning, delivery and evaluation.

EMPOWERMENT AND EMANCIPATION

Questioning dominant ideologies

The questioning of dominant ideologies can be a starting point for changing power relations. This involves the detailed critical scrutiny of taken-for-granted assumptions and beliefs about people, society and social issues. As McLeod states:

> Often the first steps in initiating change involve not direct action but creating a framework for understanding what is happening, and how things might be different. (1998a, p. 256)

Let's return first to essentialism as any way of thinking about human beings and social issues which suggests that behaviour can be attributed to 'essences' or fixed qualities. In the whole arena of social divisions and differences, social constructions can have real effects. It can be argued that essentialist discourses legitimate inequality (Thompson 1998). Differences between people are seen as natural and, therefore, grounds for inequality. Fuss explains:

> For the essentialist, the natural provides the raw material and determinative starting point for the practices and laws of the social. For example, sexual difference (the division into 'male' and 'female') is taken as prior to social differences which are mapped on to, a posteriori, the biological subject. (1989, p. 15)

Saraga (1998) argues, summarizing Hughes (1998), that essentialism implies both the permanence of a condition or identity and the homogenity of people defined by this characteristic. She analyzes a number of examples including sexual preference, ethnic minorities and disability. Of the last of these she writes:

> Disability is commonly seen as an essential, and hence permanent, characteristic of people, derived from physical/biological/psychological/ cognitive traits. (1998, p. 196)

Essentialism de-politicizes. If identity and difference are essential and substantially unchanging, then they are not amenable to being changed by political methods (Gilroy 1997).

It is possible to suggest, then, some grounds for anti-essentialism: to depathologize homosexuality, respond to the values, needs and experiences of people from different religious and cultural backgrounds, and recognize disability as a condition of a society dominated by the needs and interests of non-disabled people.

Empowerment

The term empowerment has many meanings and, as Gomm suggests, has become something of a buzz word, used differently in different contexts by different people towards their own ends. He writes:

> What can we do with a term which on the right of politics can mean privatising public services, and on the far left can mean abolishing private services; which can mean all things to all men, and something different again to some women? (1993, p. 6)

In relation to principles, empowerment within our model of enabling relationships is not a gift of the powerful to the powerless. It is taken rather than given and is always social as well as personal. Defining empowerment, Thompson is succinct:

> We can identify its core element as a process of helping people gain greater control over their lives and the sociopolitical and existential challenges they face. (1998, p. 211)

Empowerment in this sense is a challenge to professionals and the power structures of the provision of services. Hugman provides a detailed analysis and states:

> If power is not an isolated element of social life, but one which inter-weaves occupational and organisational structures with the actions of professionals, individually and collectively, then it must be examined in terms of the contexts within which the caring professions are structured and operate. (1991, p. 38)

Davey, amongst others, looks towards a broader framework:

> Empowerment must address all their problems together if it is to be meaningful. Poverty, poor housing and the nature of the social security system put a strain on relationships and lead to widespread demoral-isation. Depending on the circumstances of individuals they can lead to physical and mental ill health, criminality, addiction and the perse-cution of individual or collective scapegoats: racism, sexism, picking on individuals. (1999, p. 37)

Problems are seen as having social origins: poverty, bad housing, unremitting child care and care of old people without adequate support. Growth and change is seen as being fostered in non-hierarchical and co-operative relationships in which differences are accepted and, indeed, celebrated. Such relationships pro-vide a safe and supportive space for people to explore and express their feelings and thoughts, and to come to their own understandings of the oppression faced through the inequalities and hierarchies in society. This empowers people, in principle at least, to contribute to the transforming of hierarchical relationships and, thus, the changing of society. Standing, a physiotherapist working with people with learning difficulties, writes of the possibilities for empowerment through working in partnership with clients. She states:

> Empowerment is likely to be achieved in situations and within pro-grammes where professionals are not the key actors. The cognitive, motivational and personality changes experienced by those who gain a sense of control are the essence of empowerment. (1999, p. 256)

Barnes & Bowl also define empowerment in terms of broad ranging transfor-mations in people's lives. Their list includes: personal growth and development, gaining greater control over life choices, resistance to and subversion of dom-inant discourses and practices, a means of achieving structural change (reducing inequalities), and a process of developing and valuing different knowledges – linking knowledge and action – praxis (2001, p. 25).

Dalrymple & Burke (1995) provide a list of principles and assumptions of empowerment that have relevance across all professions. Slightly reworded, these include: empowerment is a collaborative process; the empowering process views the client as competent and capable; clients must first perceive themselves as able to effect change; competence is acquired or refined through life experiences; solutions are necessarily diverse; and informal social networks are a significant source of support.

Emancipatory practice

Moving finally in the framework to emancipatory practice, we use this term to refer to a broad arena in which a number of terms have become prominent, notably anti-discriminatory practice, anti-oppressive practice and empowerment, sometimes used interchangeably and sometimes with significantly different connotations. The term emancipatory practice is used here to encompass what can be thought of as both anti-discriminatory and anti-oppressive practice. In principle, it is about challenging inequalities in delivery and access to services, and also about changes in power relations and structures that maintain inequalities and oppression (Braye & Preston-Shoot 1995). Emancipatory practice seeks to break down walls of discrimination and to remove barriers to full participative citizenship for all.

Anti-discriminatory and anti-oppressive practice are often used as umbrella notions that incorporate challenging dominant ideologies and strategies for empowerment. Braye & Preston-Shoot (1995) differentiate between anti-discriminatory and anti-oppressive practice, highlighting some of the issues. In their model, anti-discriminatory practice is reformist, and challenges inequality within officially sanctioned rules, procedures and structures. Specific strategies include: equal access to services, ethnically sensitive services, and consultation about services. Anti-oppressive practice, in this model, seeks more fundamental changes in power structures and specific strategies include: rebalancing power relationships between professionals and clients, with client control of services and resources; and identification and challenging of abuses of power experienced by clients. The two terms, however, are often used interchangeably.

Writing of the second pillar of critical practice (deemed empowerment, though incorporating anti-oppression and anti-discrimination), Brechin points to:

> A recognition that less powerful or minority groups tend to become oppressed and disadvantaged and that health and social care services and professionals are so much a part of the status quo that they inevitably and unconsciously play a part in this structured oppression. In recognising this, critical practitioners begin to understand oppressive forces and work to reconstruct power imbalances. (2000, pp. 37–38)

Thompson (2000) has argued that good practice must take account of oppression and discrimination.

Reflections

Does the organization where you work (or where you are a student) have policies on equality of opportunity and/or anti-discrimination? If so, to what extent and in what ways do you think they are put into practice and in what ways are they simply rhetorical statements? Have you personally experienced discrimination or oppression? How might you use this experience positively to develop emancipatory practice?

Are there problems with this analysis of emancipatory practice? It can be argued that it polarizes people according to particular attributes, such as gender, ethnicity, sexuality and so on. As we saw in Chapter 5, identity can be seen as fractured, multi-layered, plural and continuously constructed across different relationships and social contexts. For Brechin, this places empowerment 'within a wider project of critical practice aiming to facilitate more permeable boundaries, acknowledge more flexible roles and identities and develop more dialogic ways of working with others' (2000, p. 41). Similarly in this framework, emancipatory practice is part of the wider project of enabling relationships, alongside critical reflection. The bridge provided between principles into practice is tenuous and debatable, laced with tensions, contradictions and dilemmas. There is a tension between promoting positive and sensitive practice, which opposes all forms of oppression, and at the same time resisting essentialism and not homogenizing the needs and aspirations of clients.

The following three general principles complete this section on enabling relationships:

1. To facilitate the recognition and questioning of power relations, structures and ideologies that limit people's freedom.
2. To promote people's prediction and control over decision-making processes that shape their lives.
3. To promote people's struggles against repression and 'man-made' sufferings, and support the removal of barriers to equal opportunities and promote full participatory citizenship for all.

Reflections

Establishing principles for enabling relationships in therapy practice is not a matter of accepting and applying someone else's principles. This would run counter to the critical reflection approach adopted in this book.

The following are the principles for enabling relationships suggested in this chapter:

1. To promote understanding of self and others through personal reflection and through dialogue.
2. To facilitate functional reflection through critical examination of the practice/process of therapy to reveal its assumptions, values and biases.
3. To develop disciplinary reflection and a critical stance towards therapy within broader debates about theory and practice.
4. To promote mutual understanding and awareness of others' preferences, wishes and needs through open two-way communication.
5. To facilitate, through working in partnership, a collaborative approach to service organization, planning, delivery and evaluation.
6. To facilitate the recognition and questioning of power relations, structures and ideologies that limit people's freedom.

(Continued)

Reflections — continued

7. To promote people's prediction and control over decision-making processes that shape their lives.
8. To promote people's struggles against repression and 'man-made' sufferings, and support the removal of barriers to equal opportunities and promote full participatory citizenship for all.

These principles need themselves to be critically scrutinized. Do they apply to all therapists and clients of any age, gender, ethnicity, race, culture, socio-economic status, sexual orientation and life circumstances? Are they in accord with your own principles in your work as a therapist? Do they provide grounds for processes of helping that are appropriate to clients who come from a wide diversity of backgrounds with values that can differ radically from your own?

It is important for you to set your own principles for enabling relationships through therapy. Look again at the eight principles listed above. Are there any you might leave out and why? Are there any you would want to reword and why? Are there any statements of principle that you see as important and that are not included in this list? On what basis do you found your principles? Are they evidence-based, based on personal or professional values, derived from practice and/or experiences of therapy from the viewpoint of clients?

PART 3

In Practice

Part 3 is based around illustrative examples of health and social care in therapy practice. The opening chapter is by Sally French and is based upon six interviews conducted with clients who have experienced considerable contact with physiotherapists, occupational therapists, and speech and language therapists in recent times. She reports on what clients value in therapists, criticisms they have, and she looks towards reflecting on and improving practice from the perspectives of clients. It is from this point of view that Sally examines processes of enabling relationships in putting principles into practice. In the following chapter Frances Reynolds considers effective two-way communication between individual therapists and clients. She begins with a detailed case study, analyzing barriers to communication, which she picks up and develops through the chapter. Frances looks at processes of building a working alliance and effective two-way communication in the therapy and rehabilitation context including: listening to the client's story, providing information, asking questions, providing feedback about progress and helping the client to manage negative thinking, supporting client's decision-making and control, and self-expression through narrative and art. Chapter 9, which is about enabling relationships in group contexts, is also by Frances. She argues that, and shows how, groups can provide the most enabling and the most inhibiting of contexts in which to communicate. She looks at the processes within groups that have many different purposes and structures, and at groups that are led by therapists/health professionals, and those that are led by clients. Through examples of groupwork in health and social care, Frances examines common barriers to enabling communications in a group context and suggestions for leading educational, remedial and supportive groups in ways that are enabling rather than disabling. In the final chapter of Part 3, John Swain turns to challenging the walls of discrimination. He explores the possibilities for change through dismantling institutional discrimination and possible strategies of professional support for change. The framework for this chapter is the same as the framework of principles offered in Chapter 6 and concentrates on: questioning dominant ideologies, empowerment and emancipatory practice.

Chapter 7

Enabling relationships in therapy practice

Sally French

This chapter is based upon six interviews that I conducted with four women, Turid, Sue, Kate and Sandy, and two men, Kevin and Harry, who have experienced considerable contact with physiotherapists, occupational therapists, and speech and language therapists in recent times. Although this sample cannot be regarded as representative of the client population, I hope it will illustrate some of the attributes clients value in therapists and some of the problems that may arise in therapist–client interaction.

WHAT DO CLIENTS VALUE IN THERAPISTS?

One of the prominent themes that emerged from these interviews was the value of therapists linking their treatment to the client's own interests and lifestyle. Turid, who has aphasia following a stroke, spoke about the value of finding common interests with her speech and language therapist:

> The therapist came from Australia, and my daughter lives in Australia and that was very nice, somehow. She asked me what animals did I know and I couldn't think of any animals except the Australian ones – kangaroos! I saw her for about six months and I got much better but she told me I wouldn't ever be able to talk properly. It was good to talk about Australia together.

Sue valued the way in which her speech and language therapist explained everything carefully and linked the treatment with her lifestyle and experience:

> The speech therapist was a very special type of person and she gave me a sense that I was being valued as a person. She listened and she gave me the answers that I was looking for. She built up my confidence

Reflections

From your experience of working with clients as a therapist or therapy student, what attributes do you think clients value most in you as a therapist?

somehow. What she did was tell me why she was doing therapy and what it was meant to achieve and she explained the purpose of what she was doing. Instead of the normal speech therapy scenarios that you would expect, she would try to connect it to my previous work as a manager so that I could relate to it. I felt she understood where I was coming from. That way I felt more in control and that gave me confidence in her as a therapist and in myself – it built up my self-confidence.

Brown & Weston believe that effective client care requires attending to the client's personal experience of illness and '... understanding the person and the world in which he or she lives' (1995, p. 44).

Kate spoke of how an occupational therapist had helped her to cope with sudden and unexpected retirement from a busy job by means of a personal diary. She linked the success of this encounter to the occupational therapist's recognition of her as a unique person:

When I gave up work, and I was very, very involved in my work, my GP referred me to occupational therapy to try and get me to come to terms with it. They were very helpful. We set up a plan together. I was filling my time with hobbies and I was driven to finish every single task all the time just as if I was at work. We explored that together. They were very supportive and very helpful. They seemed to understand what I was feeling and we made very small goals. I kept a diary that we explored and worked from. It was very positive and made a big difference.

Sue and Sandy both talked about their need for control and how the sensitivity of their physiotherapists had enabled this to happen. Sue talked of her time as an outpatient:

She said 'Come in when you like and use all the equipment'. I was particularly lucky with my physio because she had the foresight to realise that that was what I needed for my recovery – to be in control .. . She treated me like a person. She spoke to me like a person and not a patient. I felt in control and that gave me more confidence in myself. You know, having a stroke takes everything away from you very suddenly. All the time I was fighting to regain control of something, it doesn't matter what it is at first . . . I think there's a very close relationship between control and confidence – I'm sure there is – and she understood that.

Sandy was given control by the assertion of her physiotherapist, Mary, immediately after major surgery:

She said to the chief nurse 'Why is Sandy on that bed?'. She was very assertive. Some physios wouldn't have bothered. Within a short space of time these porters came with this very fancy bed that was electrically controlled by a button, you could move it into all different positions. So I didn't need my hands and arms, it meant I could move my body to places by moving the bed. I was really empowered by that bed and Mary did that and I think if Mary hadn't been who she was I would have spent the rest of my stay flat. Without that bed I'd have been in the position of saying 'I want to read now' or 'I want to lie down now' – all day and all night. That would have been horrible. That bed not only gave me control but it was very comfortable and it helped with the pain.

Harry, who used the equipment in the physiotherapy department when his rehabilitation was complete, remembered the help he was given by a physiotherapist:

I was in the physiotherapy department. They all knew me well. I was part of the furniture, and I remember saying to one of the physios, 'Why isn't there any counselling?' I said, 'There really should be counselling offered to people who've had strokes and who have communication problems.' I was doing a lot of moaning at that time because I was miserable and this physio said, 'Harry, I'm fed up with you moaning about this. I agree with you entirely but why don't you do something about it? Why don't you do a counselling course because I think you'd be really good at it?' She said, 'there's a real need for it and you have the personal qualities and experience to do it so stop moaning and do something about it.' I wandered around for weeks afterwards thinking 'I wonder' and 'maybe'. The thing that helped me so much was her belief that I could do it.

Harry is now a fully qualified counsellor and works with people with aphasia.

Emotional support and simple, effective advice was also highly valued. Kate spoke of a physiotherapist who came to treat her when she was having breathing difficulties:

It was one particular physiotherapist who came in the middle of the night and she was so helpful and made such a difference. She said, 'Try dropping your shoulders a little bit' and 'If you put a pillow in the back of your neck that will help.' I use the techniques all the time now, it seems a very small thing but it made a huge difference. On the whole physiotherapists back away because they think they can't do anything, whereas she approached it in a very different way. She realised that she didn't have to have 'hands on' at all, that is was something I could do for myself. It made an enormous difference. They are usually very physical and you are supposed to be very physical. It was a small suggestion together with emotional support. The attitude is usually 'We can't rehabilitate you so what's the point?' I'm sure most of them feel that they could use their time better.

Respect, kindness, honesty, equality and practical expertise were also highly valued. Harry said:

I liked my speech therapist. She was trying to improve my communication and I remember thinking, 'what a fantastic woman, what a fantastic job' . . . She showed kindness. Kindness is something that is not acknowledged enough. She was gentle and empathetic, I felt as if she was joining in with my struggle.

Sandy, talking of her physiotherapist, said:

> When she came to see me first of all she told me her name and that's nice, not like 'I'm the physio' which I've had before. She said 'I'm Mary' and very quickly moved into 'how are you feeling?' – not a straight 'I'm here to do.' She had a really warm manner with her and she said, 'Can I sit on the edge, is it all right?' – she didn't make assumptions. She checked that my morphine bracelet was working – all those sorts of things. She really acknowledged what I had been through, how I was feeling and a bit of a warning that the pain would be bad even with the morphine but that there would be a time when it would calm – and I call that respect because there's no denial, it's nice and straight and I value that. I value the information. Mary was concerned with strength and function so I had to do very simple things the first time. She said, 'Do the push' and I pushed and I couldn't. I was shocked. I wasn't at all prepared because before I went to sleep for that op I could push myself up with my hands. I lay back down again and I was terribly upset and I had a bit of a panic. She was lovely. She said, 'We've done the neurological tests and this is a mixture of post-op weakness and genuine loss most of which we can regain.' So I took another breath. She was very honest but she was also very tender. There was something about her presence and her being. I got to know her as a person in a very short time. She was definitely 'Mary' and not a physio.

Harry talked about the way in which his speech and language therapist accepted an outburst of frustration and anger:

> One day I went to see her and I felt terrible, very vulnerable, very low self-esteem. I remember wheeling myself into her room and with the good hand I swept everything off her desk on to the floor, the phone and everything, a big drama . . . She allowed me to get upset, I was allowed to cry and she was fantastic. She wasn't all, 'there, there, here's a hankie' and I poured it all out with broken words. She let me leave without the treatment and I just felt so much lighter, so much better . . . She didn't try to pacify me or comfort me, but I didn't want that, I wanted someone to hear me. I trusted her enough to get upset in front of her. I couldn't say what I wanted to say because I didn't have enough speech.

The people that I interviewed valued an honest, open, warm and supportive relationship with their therapists. Practical expertise was important, but so was empathy, equality and a willingness to work in partnership. They valued the ability of therapists to connect with them as unique individuals, to be assertive on their behalf and to link therapy with their interests and lifestyle. Pound, a disabled speech and language therapist, states:

> I have no doubt, that were I to become aphasic, I would seek the best aphasia therapist possible to help me improve my language skills. But in retrospect I realise that this form of expertise alone did not move me forward. I valued the careful listening of therapists and non-therapists, and the challenge to view things differently from people who lived with disabilities themselves. (In press)

Reflections

Were the attributes you considered to be important in yourself as a therapist similar to those mentioned by the people who were interviewed? Note down anything that surprised you about what they said. With a long-term client, discuss what he or she feels has been particularly helpful about his or her encounters with therapists.

WHAT CRITICISMS DO CLIENTS MAKE OF THERAPISTS?

Poor interpersonal skills and a reluctance by therapists to share power, rather than lack of technical expertise, were the dominant criticisms given by the people I interviewed. Turid explained how her treatment in speech and language therapy focused around an activity that she disliked and how wider concerns were not addressed:

> There is certain things I don't like and that is *Scrabble*. I don't like *Scrabble* – never did. I realised it was quite good for me but the thought that I had to do it – I hated the feeling about it. I didn't say anything. I thought that as I can't talk or read properly perhaps *Scrabble* is as far as I can manage. It took a long time. I used to read to sleep and then I couldn't do it and that was so upsetting, that I couldn't even read, so I listened to the music but that meant that my husband couldn't . . . he and me we couldn't sleep together so that . . . well she just talked about things like *Scrabble*. I know some people love *Scrabble*.

Sandy and Sue spoke of their experiences of occupational therapy:

> I've often thought about OTs in rehab, if only they could think about the context from which their patients came. I was received as head of department of a girls' comprehensive school, head of physical education, and this OT said to me, 'Now you've really got to learn to type because that's what you'll be doing.' She negated the whole context of my professional life – I was just a patient. Just because someone has had an accident or an illness doesn't mean that they've changed one iota. I went in as a gymnast and a sports person, that hadn't changed, it was just that I couldn't do it anymore. There was no acknowledgement of what my life was about or how to shape my new future. They had a routine. It was almost like, 'She's got fingers, she can type.' I couldn't identify with it, there was no link with anything to do with me. (Sandy)

> It was a case of being treated like a patient. I felt like my feelings were being ignored, that they were just going through a routine and they would give me exercises to do which I couldn't understand the purpose of because they didn't explain. I had enough speech to ask, but I didn't ask, because I didn't have the confidence to ask. (Sue)

Reflections

Kate gave a detailed account of the occupational therapist's failure to communicate with her about the home adaptations she required. Read the account and make a summary of Kate's complaints:

> What I did find incredibly difficult to come to terms with was somebody coming into my home and saying, 'This needs to be done and this is how it's going to be done.' I had no say whatsoever to the point where ... well one of the things is the front door which is completely flat because I'm in a wheelchair. I could cope with a small rise very easily and I demonstrated that I could manage. What happens now is that whenever you open the door the leaves blow in because it's so flat. I had quite a long argument, added to which the builder had difficulty finding such a flat front door.
>
> The other thing is the front lounge, it was designed without any discussion. I couldn't deviate from it one millimetre. It was designed as an adaptation without any thought to the fact that it was affecting my home and that it wasn't just me that it affected.
>
> The only battle that I won, and it was a major argument that held up all the work for about three months, was that they wanted to lower all the work tops in the kitchen to my height and I kept pointing out that there were three other members of the family and I didn't want to have to do all the work! What we actually did was a carpenter friend of mine put roll-out tops under the existing tops so I have something my height and they've got something at their height. It was as if I was living on my own and that the property was theirs.
>
> The other major argument I had was that initially they weren't going to put a stair lift in at all (Kate has a ground floor and a basement). They said I could live on the top level. I pointed out that I had two teenage daughters who would be completely cut off from me and I wanted to know what was going on down there. It was partly expense but they weren't looking at me holistically at all. I did get the stair lift but it wasn't done in the first wave, it was an ongoing argument. She just came in, there was no awareness of me as a person, it was a practical issue – we had to get a wheelchair around this building. But I'm a person – it's not a wheelchair that has to go through that door it's me!

Harry spoke of a physiotherapist who appeared to be avoiding communication with his patients as well as showing a total lack of empathy:

> I didn't like him. He was arrogant. He reminded me of a plate spinner – he always had about three clients on the go, he wasn't giving any of them his attention. It was only him that worked like that. Then one day his attention was diverted and this guy he was treating fell and hit the floor heavily and the physiotherapist turned round and said, 'Oh God!

Get up, come on now'. He enraged me. I tried to talk but all my speech had gone. He really upset me – it's making me feel upset talking about it now. He was just awful.

Brown & Weston remind us that clients are multi-dimensional, that they are ' . . . parents, partners, sons and daughters who have a past, a present and a future' (1995, p. 45).

Sandy found her occupational therapist distant and inflexible and was helped by a friend and her carer when the equipment from the occupational therapist could not be used:

> When I got home the social service OT came and she started as if it was day one with a big assessment when I'd had the whole thing done in hospital. I was ill and in a lot of pain, sick most of the time, couldn't eat, and I couldn't be doing with it. I thought, 'Just go away, just go to the hospital and they'll tell you everything you want to know.' She was neutral. She was just doing her job with her clipboard. I can't remember her name – she was just a professional. She came back to say that there was a waiting list for this bath thing so I'd have to have bed baths for three months from the carer. Finally this thing arrived, none of us knew it was coming, it came with a man in a van – a lovely, friendly man with this contraption – but it didn't fit. We got to 'breaking rule time' then which meant 'blow what they said'. My friend and my carer got these two boards and they made a slide system to the bath. The OT didn't help one bit. When we told her the contraption wouldn't work she said, 'Well, that's that then, it will have to be bed baths.' She never came again.

Kevin objects to going through occupational therapists for the equipment he needs:

> If you want a spade to dig your garden you don't go to an OT do you? You go down the hardware shop and buy a spade, the one that suits you. So why can't I go down to my local hardware shop and buy a button-hook, or buy a stick, or buy anything? – a tool is a tool.

Lack of communication between therapists was also cited as a difficulty. Kate said:

> Another problem is the lack of liaison between occupational therapists in the community and in the hospital. I had multiple problems, they don't talk to each other. One would promise me one thing, the next would say that I couldn't have it and another would modify it. It's very, very confusing because you really don't know what's going to happen.

Turid, on the other hand, found that the mix of different therapists helped to reduce the isolation she felt:

> I had lots of different people . . . it was OK . . . it was nice to have a mixture of people. When I first had the stroke lots of people came to see me but after two months they don't come anymore. It was quite nice to go and do all the things I had to do with my shoulders. It was nice to see different people.

Finlay (2000) emphasizes the distress that duplication can cause service users as it may appear that professionals have not listened to their previous accounts and that they are not collaborating with each other.

Kate felt that professionals tend to focus too much on their narrow, technical expertise:

> The occupational therapy assistants tend to be better. They tend to be much more aware of the person. They're much more concerned about the person's needs. I had a lovely occupational therapy assistant who I still have some contact with but I'm not on her caseload any more. When the occupational therapist took over she wasn't supposed to come any more and the change was very, very marked. It went from person-centred to technical. My husband was very resistant to any adaptation but she (the assistant) managed to get round him, she was much more aware of relationships than the qualified OT.

Pound emphasizes the importance of the non-technical aspects of the client–therapist relationship. Talking of speech and language therapists she states:

> Listening to clients discussing their likes and dislikes of individual therapy, it is often difficult to find features which relate to more technical aspects of language exercises. Most often they highlight time, space and a listening relationship as the features of therapy which they most value. It is this intense and rather intimate relationship that acts as a rock in a time of stormy chaos. It is this holding ground that becomes the first real reference point to a clearer direction and a more hopeful future. That is not to undervalue the technical skills of the therapist but it is also not to make light of the benefits of listening, respect and mutual engagement. (In press)

Reflections

It is never easy to hear ourselves criticized, especially by people we are trying to help. It can, however, be invaluable in improving practice even within the confines or constraints such as time and lack of resources. With one or two trusted colleagues read the quotations again and list the major criticisms made by the people who were interviewed. Discuss ways in which practice could be improved by taking these criticisms into account.

Disabled people who employ their own assistants, frequently avoid 'experts' preferring to train people on their own terms and in their own way (Morris 2001).

Kevin found that his relationship with his physiotherapist was unequal as he was expected to take her advice and she failed to understand his priorities:

> About two years ago I realised that my walking ability had deteriorated . . . so I talked to my GP who referred me to the physiotherapy department at my local hospital. She said, 'We can stop the deterioration provided you're willing to spend an hour a day working at it' and she didn't like it because I said I didn't feel that the work was worth it. I told her that I've got limited energy, some of my functions are not automatic, like when I'm talking I'm also trying to remember to swallow my saliva. When I'm walking I'm thinking 'left foot, right foot, left foot, right foot'. All those things are tiring. I said to her that I'm more interested in doing things that engage my mind and imagination, I'm not going to waste my energy going 'up down, up down'. She didn't like it and she wrote me off as somebody she couldn't help rather than treating me as somebody she had helped by giving me some advice.

He contrasted this with his contact with an occupational therapist:

> I worked with a very good OT at D (an organisation run by disabled people) who agreed with our philosophy. If people came she gave them advice but she had no hang-ups about whether they took it or not.

WHAT ADVICE DO CLIENTS HAVE FOR THERAPISTS?

Various pieces of advice were offered to therapists by the people I interviewed. Sue said:

> Forget you're a therapist – just be yourself. I don't mean forget all your training – but be yourself. Don't be afraid of showing the real you because that's what makes people respond, when they're ill they respond more easily if the therapist is being real.

Kate wants therapists to stop focusing on 'normality', to be flexible and to take the client's perspective into account:

> What concerns me most of all is this focus on trying to make me 'normal'. I get that from all the therapists. I get a lot of referrals of 'this may help' and 'that may help'. They had a massive case conference before the adaptations – it was a case of 'how normal can we make her first? Are the adaptations necessary?' They deliberately didn't widen the bathroom door upstairs to try and make me walk to the toilet. I very deliberately leave the feet off my wheelchair to keep my legs moving – it's definitely helped to maintain the muscle tone – but they don't like this. I can't feel them so I have to be very careful as I've been known to run over my own feet. They don't like it for safety reasons, but you make

choices – I go sailing and that could be dangerous. . . . Nobody thinks about the real world, it's all very purist. I want therapists to be flexible and realistic. I want them to say, 'What sorts of things would help you to lead a full life in the context of your impairment?' It's either, 'you're disabled and what can we do to make you better' or 'you're OK'. Nobody says 'What would make a better life?' That's what I would like.

Kevin, looking back on his school days, also feels that striving for 'normality' can be misplaced:

I remember speech therapy being a lot of hard work and I can remember getting extremely fed up. I got to a situation where I hated eating because at every mealtime the speech therapist would come into the dining room to supervise us saying, 'remember what we talked about, remember about your swallowing, remember how to drink' . . . Ok it's good to do it while you're actually eating something, rather than talking about it in theory, but when you're doing it at every mealtime, and your parents have been told so they do it at home, you get to a point when you think 'wouldn't it be nice to just sit and enjoy your food!?' You get to a point where you've eaten a meal and you can't remember what you've eaten – it becomes a technical exercise. Obviously it helped, although I still make a mess, but you've got to question it. I do question the years of not enjoying food and getting to a point when I dreaded mealtimes. But now I think, 'This is me. This is what I do. I've made a mess on my shirt and I don't give a toss. It can be cleaned up. Just eat for the pleasure of eating and to hell with the rest.' A by-product of too much therapy and too much intervention is that you go through a period when you're scared of your own shadow, but then you reach a point when you say 'tough'! If I spill my coffee I'm now more interested in the pretty pattern it makes.

Sandy wants her expertise recognized:

The biggest thing is about asking and not telling. They need to get into the habit of asking what would be helpful. They don't seem to enter into a dialogue – we respect them far more if we can have an equal partnership in the challenge we're both facing. I would expect a person to be trained to the task and have an excellent knowledge base, and I would expect to have an exchange of knowledge – theirs would be knowledge from their training and mine would be about my own body, and my lifestyle. I would expect the therapist to hear me. I would expect them to be creative.

Brown (2000) states that clients have challenged the appropriateness of professional knowledge. One way that they have done this is by insisting that their own knowledge, of illness, impairment and disability is equally as valid as that of professionals (French & Swain 2001). As Pound states:

For me, another key milestone in acknowledging my strength and experience as a disabled person was the recognition that through my experience I had acquired an expertise that my doctors and therapists lacked and that I really could make a contribution. However for many years the uncertainty with which I experienced each day was no match for the clarity and certainty of medicine and consequently I afforded it little value or status. (In press)

Harry urges therapists to develop their communication skills and to be kind:

Being kind is so important and being able to understand. I used to look at the nurses and doctors walking around and I used to think to myself, 'I could do that two weeks ago, I could walk up and down, I could talk'. It's such a shock and it's so nice when somebody at least tries to understand how you might be feeling. And I think that kindness is such a nice quality to have. It's a lovely, wonderful thing, being kind.

The people I interviewed were sympathetic towards therapists and the conditions under which they sometimes work. Turid found communication unsatisfactory on occasions but, as an older person, she can empathize with how young therapists might feel:

I can understand them, I'm nearly close to 70, and I can understand the young person who is trying to do whatever she wants to do, what she thinks is best – she's trying very hard – she's a young person. Sometimes if they try to tell people what's what, you just have to wait – and it goes. Some of them might be a bit frightened of me because I'm older – it might scare them. That's what I think – but that might be my fantasy.

Sandy could empathize with the conditions under which therapists work:

Creativity is a big thing and sadly because of time constraints and budgetary constraints some therapists have their creativity stifled. The systems don't help therapists to be creative and relaxed. The hospital OT seemed more ordinary and more creative. She was a lovely, relaxed person. The community one wasn't really concerned with me, she was doing her job. The approach was colder – it was a business approach rather than a human connection. Perhaps the community ones are more isolated and not supported. I've been in situations like that myself and I know how it feels.

Kevin could understand the difficulty of working in organizations but urges therapists to keep to their principles:

When you leave education, when you've got your qualification, be aware that the people you work for will try and make you conform to the traditional way of working. You may need to do that initially, but try not to allow yourself to become corrupted by it. Keep your integrity because when you get a bit higher up the ladder, and get a bit of power, you can try to change things.

He also believes that therapists need to relinquish their power and that fundamental changes are needed in therapy education and practice:

> Users should have more power. Until you give users real power, real control we'll get nowhere . . . there's an awful lot of people with a lot of vested interests. The more we shout about rights the more people get afraid. I'd like to see therapy training following the social model rather than the medical model. The only way to do it is to get much more input from disabled people into the training. It would be a national scandal if men did a whole load of training on women's issues, it would be unheard of for a group of white people to give equality training on race, but medical people do their training without coming up against it, without being challenged . . . Let's get away from the medical model, not only in training, but in practice. Let's get a divorce between the medical profession and therapists. Let's get them out from social services as independent professionals with skills and knowledge . . . they're in a hierarchy and the doctors don't want to let go.

The advice given in these interviews is similar to that of Stewart & Weston who advocate practice that is patient-centred. They state:

> The patient-centred model of care presupposes a change in the mind-set of the clinician. The hierarchical notion of the professional being in charge and the patient being passive does not hold here. To be patient-centred the practitioner must be able to empower the patient, to share the power in the relationship; this means reducing control which has traditionally been in the hands of the professional. (1995, p. xvi)

Pound (In press) advises therapists to: frequently acknowledge the client's expertise and not overpower clients with their own expertise; value the impact of authentic and responsive listening; ensure that any theory or advice given is accessible; and exploit fun and creativity in therapy.

Reflections

Read these quotations again and jot down all the pieces of advice that the people I interviewed offered. How far do you agree with them? With one or two trusted colleagues consider ways in which you could use their advice to improve practice, despite the constraints under which you may work.

CONCLUSION

By means of a few interviews and a brief exploration of the relevant literature, this chapter has highlighted the views and experiences of clients regarding their relationships with therapists. Clients value the technical expertise of therapists but focus more on their interpersonal qualities valuing warmth, realism, flexibility, genuineness, honesty, kindness and the ability to share power and to work in partnership. Without these qualities therapy interventions are unlikely to succeed, as success is dependent on engaging with the clients' ideas, feelings, aspirations, expectations and lifestyle, and recognizing their own expertise.

Chapter **8**

Two-way communication

Frances Reynolds

This chapter will explore some of the skills and attitudes that assist therapists to establish a partnership, or working alliance, with their clients and patients. It has been argued in previous chapters that many barriers to genuine partnership are set in place by conceptual and organizational factors. Even though these external constraints exist, the skills and attitudes of the individual therapist are, nevertheless, important co-determinants of the quality of enabling interactions. With this in mind, the chapter considers effective two-way communication between individual therapists and clients.

Reflections

Consider the case study below. What barriers do you perceive to effective partnership between the client and his therapists?

Mr Ken Walker was a self-employed builder, aged 55 years. Married since his early 20s, with two sons, who worked with him in his business, he regarded himself as a successful 'self-made' man. His life changed radically one day when he experienced a stroke (CVA). As a result of the stroke, Ken's mobility was affected. The right side of his body felt weak and he had limited fine control over his dominant right hand. He was somewhat dysarthric (having limited control over the muscles involved in speech). He spent 6 weeks in a stroke rehabilitation unit. During his time there, Mr Walker was sometimes tearful. When not evidently upset, he tended to be quiet and unco-operative. He quite often referred to darkness, and repeated certain phrases. 'It's coming for me. It's so dark, so dark, like a shadow'. These comments rather alarmed some of the therapists in the multi-disciplinary team, who speculated whether the stroke had resulted in psychiatric problems. One therapist when working with Mr Walker replied briskly that he was talking 'complete nonsense' whenever he referred to darkness and shadows. He also told him that he was lucky to be making such a good recovery. A more junior therapist felt very uneasy in his presence, and tended to spend minimum time with him. During therapy, she endeavoured to focus exclusively on the therapy task to avoid communicating with him about his feelings and fears.

A number of strategies for opening up communication in creative, enabling ways will be explored. Several reflective exercises are also included to increase awareness of interactive processes and to encourage further practice of interpersonal skills. Working effectively in groups is examined in the next chapter.

BUILDING A WORKING ALLIANCE IN THE THERAPY AND REHABILITATION CONTEXT

In Chapter 7, some of the key features that characterize a working alliance, or partnership, with clients/patients were presented. These features include: enabling people to have a voice and be heard; respecting the diversity of people's aspirations and values; challenging the structural, attitudinal and environmental barriers that discriminate against ill and disabled people; and enabling people to develop their own potential.

In order to address these important goals, the therapist requires a variety of skills and personal attributes. Carl Rogers proposed that therapists and counsellors need to offer clients three forms of experience, if they are to forge a client-centred working alliance (Rogers 1967). These are:

1. warmth and unconditional positive regard
2. empathy
3. genuineness or congruence.

Burnard argues that:

> . . . these personal qualities cannot be described as 'skills' but they are necessary if we are to use interpersonal skills effectively and caringly. They form the basis and bedrock of all effective human relationships. (1996, p. 45)

Warmth, empathy and genuineness seem to reflect the therapist's deeply held values rather than the superficial performance of certain interactive behaviours. They help the therapist to enter the client's subjective world without fear or judgement. They encourage an open and honest meeting between two individuals, rather than an encounter governed primarily by the role and status of each person. If the client experiences the therapist as a trusted partner in the process of confronting fears and difficulties, he/she will gain a profound form of support that enables coping, successful adaptation to changed circumstances, and the possibility of regaining or maintaining an acceptable quality of life. Furthermore, clients who experience their therapists as listening carefully and without judgement are more likely to be able to identify their own concerns, needs and goals, thereby recovering their capacity to direct their own future.

In the case example above, the therapists seem to be having difficulty in communicating all of the core conditions. Empathy seems to be in short supply as the therapists seem unable to appreciate that the client may be deeply

Reflections

Consider the three core conditions, and decide whether these seem evident in the therapists' approach to working with Mr Ken Walker. Is the client missing out on any of these therapeutic experiences?

depressed. It is possible that Mr Walker considers his world to have been turned upside down without warning by the stroke. He may fear that his resultant loss of function will threaten his livelihood and undermine his sense of himself as a successful husband and father. If he cannot work, his family's financial position may be precarious. His sense of loss may be all the greater as his sons currently work with him in the family business. He may fear for their futures also, if his business fails. To have empathy for the client would include a preparedness to consider the deeper symbolic meanings of the images that the client is describing. The 'dark shadow' may be a metaphor, perhaps for loss, despair or anxiety about the future.

The client also appears to be receiving little warmth or unconditional positive acceptance. The therapist who briskly attempts to 'jolly' the client or who dismisses the client's concerns as 'nonsense' cannot be described as conveying unconditional acceptance. Obviously, at certain times, humour can be valuable within the therapeutic relationship, but it should be introduced with some caution, and certainly should not be used primarily to increase the comfort of the therapist by smothering the client's expressions of distress. Making comparisons between the situation of the client and that of others, and the therapist's judgement (as an 'outsider') that the client is 'lucky', also shows a lack of acceptance of the person's own perspective and feelings. For a person engaged in the process of grieving, it would be more helpful to feel *heard*, rather than *judged*. It would also be appropriate for the therapists to recognize the diversity of responses among individuals who have experienced a stroke (or other illness). Some may be up-beat in their appraisal of their functioning, and positive about the possibility of achieving a good quality of life. Others, particularly in the early stages, may judge their illness to have robbed them of everything that made life worthwhile.

If they are to offer unconditional positive acceptance, therapists need above all to value their clients as people, with their own unique characteristics, strengths and vulnerabilities. Rogers termed this 'prizing'. As indicated in Chapter 2, the therapist translates this valuing into careful listening to the whole of the client's story, and not simply the biomedical details. Medically similar illnesses may have widely different meanings and implications for individuals, depending upon their social context, personal priorities and resources. In the case above, the client does not seem to receive unconditional acceptance. The therapists fail to understand his communications and instead attempt to explain his behaviour in terms of psychiatric symptoms. Whilst professional opinion may, of course, be needed to determine whether

> **Reflections**
>
> Why do you think that the therapists in this case study have certain problems in maintaining the core conditions of the working alliance? Reflect on any difficulties that you might have in maintaining empathy, unconditional acceptance or genuineness, if you were Mr Walker's therapist, and consider why difficulties might occur. Take some time reflecting on this issue, and be honest!

neurological damage is directly implicated in fantasies and emotional instability following stroke or other forms of brain injury, it is also important to resist attributing *all* discomforting reactions to brain lesions. At least one-third of individuals experience depression following stroke (as with other serious illnesses), and this can at least partially be explained in terms of a psychological response to loss of personal identity, communication difficulties and social isolation (Ellis-Hill & Horn 2000, Ellis-Hill et al. 2000, Ouimet et al. 2001).

Finally, in the case above, Ken Walker did not seem to receive a genuine or congruent response from his therapists. Therapists who respond to their own personal discomfort by focusing exclusively on the task in hand, thereby avoiding communication, are behaving incongruently. The therapist's internal emotional state is kept separate from the behaviour that is on display. Despite the intentions to hide negative emotions, the resulting avoidance behaviour is apt to betray the therapist's discomfort, increasing the client's confusion about the message being sent. The client may feel rejected or shameful as a result. The partnership would have been better served had the therapist commented more openly, perhaps admitting that she found it difficult to interpret Mr Walker's concerns, and inviting him to talk more about the dark shadow that seemed to be menacing him.

RE-VISITING SOME BARRIERS TO THE WORKING ALLIANCE

A number of cultural, organizational and professional barriers to developing partnership approaches with clients have been previously discussed in Chapter 2. These include the lengthy professional training that creates social distance between health professional and client, tending as a result to objectify the client. Rogers (1967) argued:

> I feel quite strongly that one of the important reasons for the professionalization of every field is that it helps to keep this distance . . . we develop elaborate diagnostic formulations, seeing the person as an object . . . In these ways, I believe, we can keep ourselves from experiencing the caring which would exist if we recognized the relationship as one between two persons . . . (reprinted in Kirschenbaum & Henderson 1990, p. 120).

Professional training shapes therapists' perceptions of illness. In acquiring detailed biomedical knowledge about disease processes, and from treating numerous clients daily, the therapist may lose sight of each client's own perspective. There is a range of evidence suggesting that doctors, for example, tend to extract from patients' accounts of their illness, only the details most relevant to biomedicine. 'Analysis of interchanges between doctors and their patients often show patient narratives as neglected or re-organized through the doctor's "medicalizing" discussion' (Mattingly 1998, p. 12). Yet for each individual client, illness or impairment is a uniquely personal experience, and may be interpreted variously – for example as a profound loss, as a normal state of the body, as a challenge, or as an opportunity for growth and change. Such interpretations can also change over time. The therapist needs to be aware that individual differences exist in the meanings of illness, and be highly responsive to the client's own perspective in order to work in effective partnership.

Organizational pressures, such as limited therapy time, also militate against effective partnerships, as the therapist may, understandably, feel pressurized to 'do' therapy, rather than to listen to the client's concerns. Nevertheless, it does not *necessarily* take much time to acknowledge that you have heard a client's concerns. In the case above, therapists may have feared opening up a conversation about painful issues that could not be properly explored within the scheduled therapy session. Some therapists who counsel clients in physical rehabilitation settings have commented on their fear of going in 'too deep, too soon', without the means of assisting the client to end the session in an emotionally safe place (Reynolds 1999a). They express concern that the client's feelings may be left very exposed unless there is an opportunity for sensitive closure within the therapy session, and perhaps the setting in place of further support. To accomplish effective care, it is not only the individual therapist who requires appropriate counselling skills. The whole team needs to be alert to clients' emotional distress. Ideally, some means of adjusting therapy time to the individual client's needs is required – yet this may be difficult to arrange given organizational constraints. A designated rehabilitation counsellor within the multi-disciplinary team may be desirable, to offer appropriate skills and time to clients who request additional support. However, in settings where therapists lack advanced counselling skills, whole team support, and the opportunity to refer clients on for more specialist help, it is understandable that they may simply attempt to maintain their own comfort by closing down clients' communications about emotional distress.

Therapists also sometimes avoid listening to their clients because they feel ill-equipped in terms of counselling skills, and fearful of not being able to cope with clients' concerns. Yet even therapists with advanced training in counselling skills can fear burnout, a condition characterized by emotional exhaustion and feelings of depersonalization. It can be difficult for such therapists to withstand pressures from the multi-disciplinary team to become the main source of support to distressed clients (Reynolds 1999a).

Not surprisingly, such a solitary role places a heavy emotional burden on the therapist. Whilst therapists require a high level of reflective awareness and a wide repertoire of personal communication skills to be responsive to clients' needs, they also need to be part of an emotionally literate work context that provides appropriate support, and clinical supervision for the whole team. A single team member should never be designated as the only person doing 'emotional work' with clients.

The previous discussion suggests that the barriers to effective partnership are numerous, and that effective support for therapists and clients alike depends on the wider team and organizational culture. Yet not all failures of communication are the product of a disabling social world or rigid health-care systems incapable of responding to individual needs. The attitudes and communication skills of individual therapists do make a vital contribution. Clients tend to take the technical competence of health professionals for granted and notice those who listen carefully, offer effective explanations, and so on (Gerteis et al. 1993). Therapists' communication skills can make a significant difference to clients' capacity to deal with crisis and cope with change.

The remainder of this chapter encourages you to reflect on your personal values and styles of communication and to take steps to develop your skills further. First, we will clarify what is involved in effective two-way communication, and then consider several types of communication in the therapy setting that enable clients to adapt successfully and reach their personal goals.

EFFECTIVE TWO-WAY COMMUNICATION IN THE THERAPY SETTING

As shown in Chapter 1, effective communication is never a one-way process involving a simple *transmission* of information. Successful communication means that each person in the encounter reaches a shared agreement about the message that they have *shared*. In effective two-way communication, the message 'sent' by one partner is the same as the message 'received' by the other. In the previous case example, Mr Walker 'sent' his therapists a message about his thoughts and fears, framed in terms of the metaphor of the black shadow, yet the therapists did not manage to decode his meaning, even partially. They interpreted his behaviour as a sign of psychiatric disturbance, without any genuine personal significance. Their responsiveness to the multiple, and subtle messages that the client was conveying was extremely limited.

As well as requiring effective listening skills, therapists frequently need effective skills for 'sending' messages that are straightforward for the client to interpret. Information is central to empowerment, but only if it is properly understood by the client can it enable decision-making, coping and change.

In medical and rehabilitation settings, the use of jargon tends to mystify rather than clarify. It is important for therapists to be mindful that only the

Reflections

Draw up a list of 5–10 technical terms that are a regular part of your professional vocabulary. Then consider how many of these terms are likely to be unfamiliar to clients. Plan how you might communicate the information without recourse to the specialist 'jargon', and without sounding patronizing.

most confident, assertive clients are likely to seek further information when faced with baffling explanations. Perceived power differentials result in clients rarely commenting openly on the unsuitability of the information presented. Yet both their physical safety and emotional well-being will be compromised if they leave the encounter with unanswered questions. For effective two-way communication to be achieved, the health professional needs to 'step into the client's shoes', to anticipate what information may be most needed, and then take *active* steps to seek feedback from the client, for example checking whether the client understands and is satisfied with the information given.

Therapists need a wide variety of communication skills if they are to work in enabling partnerships with clients. Without providing an exhaustive list, the most important skills include: listening and understanding the client's story; providing information; asking questions; motivating, encouraging and re-establishing hope; providing feedback about progress; helping the client to challenge negative thoughts and expectations; supporting the client's decision-making, and control; and conscientization – raising awareness of disabling cultural forces.

Although listed separately, the skills outlined need to be used together and not alone for truly two-way communication to be established. For example, the *giving* of information needs to be accompanied by a preparedness to *receive* information, in the sense of observing and checking whether the client has understood. These skills are inevitably used in combination to help clients during rehabilitation to accomplish the complex tasks of identifying meaningful goals, and finding meaning in the events that have happened to them, with the ultimate purpose of 're-authoring' their lives. Therapists and clients can be understood to be involved jointly in recreating a more positive narrative.

Reflections

Consider the many forms of interaction that occur between therapist and client in the clinical setting that you would define as 'enabling'. If possible, share your list with others to extend it. Also consider the defining characteristics of 'disabling' communications in the clinical setting.

All communications, such as listening or information-giving, involve both verbal and non-verbal channels. It is said that people are much less aware of their non-verbal communications, including facial expression, tone of voice, gestures, posture and use of space in the encounter. For this reason, non-verbal behaviour tends to 'leak' emotions and attitudes in an unedited way. Therapists need a high level of reflective awareness about their own non-verbal communications in order to understand how they might be perceived by clients. Equally, they require sensitivity to their clients' non-verbal behaviour as it will provide a rich source of clues about their emotional state, their need for information, their satisfaction with therapy and so on.

Listening to the client's story

Listening skills and responsiveness are arguably the most vital for establishing a working alliance. To listen fully to the client enables the therapist to enter the client's subjective world and to communicate an 'acceptant understanding' (Rogers 1986, p. 198). Listening and empathic understanding are central to providing the client with emotional care (Bennett 1993). Yet some disabled people comment that listening is in short supply in many rehabilitation contexts. Seymour asks:

> Are rehabilitation workers unwittingly encouraging their patients to deny the lived reality of their bodies? Are [for example] paralysed people trained to manage their bodies and adjust their lives in order to become something that others can live with?. . . In its pursuit of a 'good result', rehabilitation may neglect the person as an embodied subjectivity. (1998, p. 21)

The personal meanings that illness, impairment and transition have for the individual remain unheard. Particularly in the early stages of illness or rehabilitation, when clients are usually at their most vulnerable, it can be painful for therapists to listen in a committed way to their personal stories, and to walk beside them in a landscape that is often bleak, chaotic or frightening. Furthermore, in some exchanges, it may be difficult to interpret the client's meanings. For example, Frank (1995) gave the example of a patient who asked 'Can you give me the courage I need?' He argued that had the doctor or therapist viewed this question through a biomedical lens, it might have been interpreted simply as a sign of treatable, clinical depression. In that case, the professional 'would have missed the opening to a relationship' (Frank 1995, p. 158). Through asking this question, the patient was inviting partnership, but a health professional who concentrated on listening specifically for clues to diagnosis and biomedical treatment, would not hear this invitation.

To listen involves sustained attention to both verbal and non-verbal communications of the partner in the interaction, whilst reflectively monitoring

> **Reflections**
>
> Think of all the ways that a person in dialogue with another can reveal that he/she is not listening. List all the attitudes, skills and behaviours that contribute to attentive listening.

one's own responses. Attention is generally conveyed through use of eye contact and looking, an alert posture and an orientation towards the listener. However, a sensitive listener also respects the partner's individual and cultural needs, and adapts the listening response accordingly. For example, some clients may be comfortable with therapists who look into their face steadily whilst they are speaking, whilst others, for reasons of family or cultural background, find prolonged eye contact anxiety-provoking or disrespectful. Active listening involves suspending judgement about right and wrong, and a preparedness to attend sensitively to the client's metaphorical language, and to interpret what is *not* being said. Some disabled people have commented on the need that they have felt at some point in their lives to deny or minimize their impairments – often to gain acceptability in a disabling society (French 1993), and sometimes to preserve an 'able' self-image (Charmaz 1991). What they are *not* saying in the encounter may, therefore, provide clues to their experience of disability.

Metaphorical language seems to be quite commonly used by people undergoing trauma or transition, as it helps them to grapple with the unexpected, or disordered world in which they now live: 'Through metaphor people are able to reframe the inexplicable and reorganise their lives' (Becker 1997, p. 65). People also draw upon cultural metaphors that encompass good and evil, order and chaos, in order to gain familiarity and perhaps mastery over the adverse events that they are confronting. Metaphoric language, which draws on ideas and images available in the culture at large, can help to convey complex and unfamiliar emotions. For example, Becker (1997) recounts how some couples described their feelings about infertility, using the metaphor of the 'black hole', into which their feelings of well-being had become sucked without possibility of escape. In the case example that started this chapter, it seems likely that Ken's metaphorical use of the 'black shadow' might well have conveyed feelings about being overwhelmed by his illness or the implications that it had for him, although his therapists resisted attempting to understand these meanings. Two-way communication is more readily achieved when therapists have respect for the client's metaphorical language.

Whilst it is important for therapists to be attentive to imagery and metaphor, and to be willing to 'read between the lines', it is imperative to avoid assuming any superior knowledge about clients' hidden meanings. Some disabled people who are well adapted to their impairment have expressed exasperation that health professionals all too often assume that a positive outlook *necessarily* signifies a denial of grief about disability (e.g. Morris 1991). It is important to recognize that individuals interpret their health and life situations in many different ways. For some, not talking greatly about loss or impairment reflects acceptance; for others, it may suggest avoidance or a defensive masking of their distress. Also, living with chronic illness and or an impairment acquired in adulthood is a *process*. Some people, following an illness or accident, take time to construct a positive identity and fresh purpose in life (Thomas 1999). They tell different forms of personal story, and require different forms of support, throughout this process.

Listening is not a matter of passively soaking up information from the client. The therapist needs to be an active witness to the client's story (or testimony, see Frank 1995). Active listening also involves acknowledging what one has heard, through summarizing and paraphrasing key points back to the client, and by reflecting on what one has inferred about the emotions expressed in the communication. Such feedback in turn helps clients to feel heard and to become more aware of her/his own feelings, thoughts and goals. It emphasizes the therapist's genuine interest in the client's narrative, and helps to cement the working alliance. It also allows the client to correct the therapist's emergent understanding, helping to avoid miscommunication and conflicting agendas. Active listening contributes to empathy with the client's experience.

By listening carefully to clients, the therapist offers a number of therapeutic and empowering experiences. In summary, active listening:

- provides a witness to pain and suffering
- gives permission to express emotion
- reduces the client's sense of isolation
- increases support
- helps the client to become more aware of his/her emotional state, goals, conflicts, etc.
- acknowledges difficulties and barriers to progress openly so that they can be addressed
- brings the client's *individual* story into the open, increasing the possibility of partnership
- helps the client to situate their illness/injury in the context of their life story, to make better sense of what has happened
- assists clients in the process of creating meaning from adverse events, and to re-author their lives in a positive way. (Mattingly 1998)

Reflections

With a partner, take turns to talk and listen. Each partner takes about 5 minutes to talk about an issue with some emotional content, but one that he/she feels comfortable about disclosing. For example, 'speakers' may reflect on barriers to communication that they have personally encountered in the clinical setting, as a student, therapist or patient. For this 5 minutes, the

Reflections – continued

designated 'listener' needs to show attention, and from time to time needs to reflect back the emotional content of the speaker's disclosure, and paraphrase the main points. At the end of the encounter, the speaker might share aspects of the experience of being listened to. Did the listener really convey understanding and support? If so, how was this conveyed? Were there times when the speaker felt that the listener's attention had drifted away? Did active listening really help the speaker to clarify any thoughts and feelings about the issue in question? The 'listener' may also contribute to this reflective feedback by analyzing any positive or negative experience that arose during the exercise. Repeat the exercise, by exchanging roles.

   This exercise may seem artificial, but it begins the process of reflective awareness that can be taken forwards and developed further in the clinical setting.

Providing information

It is increasingly accepted that users of services need full information if they are going to be empowered to make decisions and gain the resources that they need to live a maximally satisfactory life. Bennett (1993) refers to this as 'informational care' and reminds therapists that they should not wait for clients to ask. Therapists are in the position to provide a wide range of information and explanation, for example about the purposes of therapy, including the rationale for specific exercises; the client's health condition/impairment; the therapy/care/medical treatment/occupational options; recommended self-help activities and regimens to carry out at home (e.g. dietary changes to control diabetes or exercises to manage back pain); the safe use of equipment/aids to daily living; local support groups and organizations; disability benefits and evidence for the efficacy of treatment.

   Providing information to clients is a challenging task for many therapists, as information will only empower if it is well understood. To be understood by clients, the therapist needs to tailor the information to the individual client and *to check how it has been received*. To do this well, the therapist may adopt the following strategies:

- Check what the client already knows.
- Invite the client to formulate questions.
- Make explanations clear and accessible without the use of unfamiliar jargon.
- Avoid a patronizing approach.
- Support the verbal explanation with written information, and diagrams whenever possible.
- Encourage the client to seek further clarification.

- Check whether the client has understood the most important points, for example by demonstrating the safe use of equipment, or by repeating the exercises that are to be carried out subsequently at home.
- Refer the client to further sources of accessible information.

In illustration, I will quote from an interview with a woman who has multiple sclerosis (MS). She took part in a project that explored women's ways of living positively with illness. Her comment revealed the difference that her physiotherapist's explanations had made to her:

> She's very, very helpful actually. She's been able to tell me what my body's doing which the doctors haven't really done. I was just in the dark before really but she's telling me, she's explaining to me about going into spasm. I had all this pain but I didn't know why before.

In order to provide empowering information, sometimes therapists have to be prepared to develop their own knowledge further. For example, if the client asks for the scientific evidence that supports a particular approach to therapy (e.g. why continuing with physical activity is now recommended to manage low back pain), it may be appropriate for the therapist to find out more about this. In turn, the client will receive a more convincing explanation for the treatment or suggested lifestyle changes rather than an empty platitude. Such knowledge will then help the client to become a more committed partner in rehabilitation. Therapists sometimes need to search out information about local resources that meet the needs of a particular client. They may also consider equipping the client with the skills to find out for himself/herself. Another interviewee with MS told me about her difficulties in finding an accessible adult education art class:

> I was offered a social services place but I thought no I don't want to do that. I've got no qualms about being disabled but I've got qualms about being locked into a corner with . . . You know I'm *me* with MS, you know, but a lot of these places, they *are* MS or whatever . . . and their identity is lost, so it's not for me.

According to this participant, health- and social-care professionals did not have any information about local community facilities, or their accessibility for a wheelchair user, and simply expected her to attend a day centre. Whilst some clients were evidently quite satisfied with this arrangement, this particular individual envisaged for herself a different leisure experience – one that the therapists seemed ill-equipped to advise about. In contrast, another interviewee with MS was very happy with the tailored advice that she had received from her occupational therapist, which had enabled her to continue with embroidery, which for her was a highly valued leisure pursuit. Increasing mobility and dexterity problems had created pain and made it difficult for the woman to sew. One therapist had simply suggested that she abandon this activity, without considering the importance of this occupation for her self-esteem and identity. Fortunately, she had received more empowering advice from another occupational therapist on positioning, seating and the use of a cushion under her arm, to enable embroidery with less strain. The therapist had also demonstrated further energy saving strategies for her client's other daily activities. The information had been genuinely 'enabling', resulting in the client being able to continue with a leisure occupation that had much meaning for her. She explained the importance of her artwork as much more than a simple time-filler:

> I find doing the embroidery gives you a little bit of dignity because I feel I can give back because I don't want to keep taking from life. I want to give as well and . . . make people happy as well by doing them a hand-made birthday card.

From her perspective, her creative work helped to maintain her active involvement in her social circle, and her ability to reciprocate the care that others were giving to her. It helped to define her 'adult' rather than 'dependent' status, which she found problematic. By taking these needs seriously, and understanding the role of embroidery in this particular woman's life, the therapist had succeeded in providing empowering information. This illustration emphasizes that providing information is not simply reliant on therapists having efficient verbal skills, but depends upon their preparedness to gain insights into the client's social worlds, and to respect their goals and priorities. Empathy and respect for disabled people may be further developed by a number of experiences, including open discussion with people who have first-hand experience of illness and impairment, reading about disabled people's own experiences – as reported in qualitative research and autobiography – and accessing the disability studies literature.

Asking questions

Questions form part of the two-way conversations that therapists frequently have with their clients. Questions can be open, inviting reflective answers, using words such as 'how', 'when', 'what', or by framing the invitation to speak with words such as 'Could you tell me about . . . ?'. The use of 'why?' should be sparing, as it tends to turn an exchange into an interrogation (Burnard 1996). Closed questions invite yes/no answers or brief statements. For example, 'do you live in a flat?' or 'when did the accident happen?'. Closed questions can be useful for gaining specific information but they direct the encounter according to the therapist's own priorities. Too many closed questions may lead to increasingly short answers, as the client makes the inference that he/she has no real power to negotiate the encounter. On the other hand, clearly the therapist needs specific information in order to work effectively with clients, so a balance of questions is usually needed. Therapists need reflective awareness of their questioning style, if they are to form an effective alliance with clients. Questions that invite the client to consider their personal response to illness or treatment, their hopes, fears, goals, ideas for tackling difficult barriers to progress, and their own resources all enable partnership. The working alliance is strengthened through opening up such topics of conversation.

Let us consider some of the common problems with therapists' questions, from the clients' viewpoint. They tend to be repetitive, with many health professionals asking the same questions and not sharing information. They tend to focus on gaining biomedical information rather than information that will place clients in the context of their wider biography. Answers to questions are all too often interrupted by the professional (Dickson et al. 1997 provide more evidence on these matters).

In summary, whilst questions can be very useful for helping the client and therapist to negotiate shared agendas, all too often they function simply to channel the interviews and assessments along lines dictated by the therapist. The interview then reflects and reinforces a model of rehabilitation that focuses narrowly on physical or functional recovery. For example, a paralyzed interviewee told Seymour that her therapists had focused on:

> . . . how I was going to manage stairs and how I was going to get to and from the bathroom. But never how I was going to look after my baby. (1998, p. 71)

On the other hand, therapists need to be aware that some clients do not wish health professionals to gain any access into their personal lives, believing that their ascribed role is to restore physical functioning. Once again, such differ-

---

Reflections

You will need a partner for this exercise. Decide who will have the main responsibility for asking the partner questions. Decide on a mutually agreed topic, and certain ground rules that prevent over-intrusive questioning. Suggested topics include your reasons for choosing to become a therapist; your first reactions to entering university or the clinical setting; a difficult choice that you have had to make.

After a 10-minute encounter, take time to reflect on the nature of the exchange. What kinds of questions were asked? Did they tend to be open, inviting reflective comment, or closed, inviting brief yes/no or one-word answers? Did the questioner impose a personal agenda, reflecting his or her own experiences and concerns in relation to the topic? Were the questions sensitively framed in response to earlier replies from the speaker? Did the questioner feel pressured to think of the next question instead of listening, or feel preoccupied with 'me too' responses? Did the 'speaker' feel as though adequate time was given to formulate a considered reply – or feel pressurized to come up quickly with a glib answer? Did the speaker feel 'enabled' to reflect on past experience, or feel constrained by the focus of the questions? Did the speaker discover an aspect of past experience that previously had been hidden?

When reactions to the exercise have been fully explored, reverse the roles and repeat the exercise. At the end, draw up some of the characteristics of skilful questioning that you have experienced.

ences in clients' stated preferences emphasize that therapists need to be flexible in their communication style.

Questions provide a central means of opening up a more holistic discussion with the client, but should generally be used sparingly. A bombardment of questions tends to close down two-way communication.

Motivating: providing feedback about progress and helping the client to manage negative thinking

Some users of services are highly motivated to make good use of available resources and to achieve their personal goals. People with long-term conditions often become experts in their own rehabilitation and strategies for living. Some individuals, however, particularly those who have experienced a sudden and unexpected failure in their health or functioning (e.g. after a stroke or spinal injury), and who are in the early stages of treatment, feel overwhelmed by negative thoughts about the future. They doubt that their identity and quality of life can ever be restored. Some are demoralized by their belief that the treatment will not have any beneficial effect. Some place the responsibility for 'curing' the condition squarely with the health professional, and do not see themselves as having any active role. For whatever reason, the therapist may have great difficulty in motivating the person to engage in the rehabilitation process, or to follow treatment recommendations. In turn, such disengagement from therapy may impede the client in learning effective strategies for managing and living with the condition, in all its physical, psychological and social aspects, and achieving personally valued goals. Therapists need a good understanding of motivational issues, as sometimes they motivate clients clumsily, for example by 'jollying' at inappropriate times, or by being patronizing.

Some of the following suggestions for helping clients regain motivation may also be relevant:

- Explore, using active listening skills, the clients' barriers to motivation, such as emotional distress, fears about the future, family pressures and role loss. This may take time, as disclosure of deeper issues requires trust and rapport.
- Be realistic and genuine with clients – they will detect false reassurances and fake jollity.
- Offer specific guidelines for any health-promoting activity that the client is advised to participate in outside of the treatment session, with written information as a support if necessary, as these are easier to follow than vague and general statements.
- Measure and record change in functioning, to provide evidence of 'objective' success – this is likely to motivate you and may be of interest to some clients.
- Encourage clients to notice *subjective* change between sessions and to record this in a diary.
- Strengthen the working alliance by inviting the clients to 'trouble-shoot' any problems arising in therapy, and to share their ideas for solving these problems.

> **Reflections**
>
> Think of a situation in which you have been poorly motivated – for example, perhaps in preparing for an examination in a subject that you disliked. Consider either what helped you to regain your motivation, or, with the benefit of hindsight, what other experiences might have been helpful? Consider whether communications with friends or family helped or hindered you in regaining motivation, and why? If possible, share your reflections with another person, and see to what extent they are similar or different.
>
> What have you learned from this activity that would help you to motivate clients in the clinical setting more appropriately?

- Support the client in repeated re-tellings of the life story, as these narratives help the person to integrate the newer and older facets of self, and to release stress.
- Assist clients to use and further develop their own sources of support, including client support organizations.
- Encourage clients to develop their own meaningful short-term and long-term goals, and to envisage the possibility of positive growth from the illness experience (but do not attempt to do this too soon, as clients who are grieving their loss of functioning may need considerable time to work through the process).

Therapists need to be sensitive to the sometimes lengthy and challenging process of coming to terms with illness, impairment and identity change. Those who live in particularly disabling environments are likely to have a harder time. For example, family or spousal criticism, or unsupportive colleagues or managers at work, may exacerbate the experience of loss and powerlessness (Schwartz & Kraft 1999). In the early stages following illness or injury, the client may benefit most from active listening and empathic communications. Later on, for those experiencing grief, communications that encourage re-engagement in activities and the development of new future plans may be more therapeutic (Worden 1983). Therapists also need to be mindful that some of their clients, particularly those who have had life-long physical impairments, regard their health or functioning as unexceptional, and as presenting no barrier to a full and active life. Their needs for enabling communications may be quite different, and may be better served in group contexts, particularly those over which users have full control.

Supporting clients' decision-making and control

Bennett (1993) argues that communications that offer clients control, as well as emotional and informational care, are a vital part of a holistic approach to therapy. The experience of illness and health care tends to undermine the client's sense of control in multiple ways (Leventhal et al. 1999, Thompson &

Kyle 2000). Illness comes unbidden into the person's life and may then proceed to steal away his/her roles and dreams. Subsequent medical treatment and hospitalization often threaten control by casting the client in a passive, dependent position. Hospital procedures, such as requiring patients to wear night clothes during daytime hours, also reinforce a subjective loss of identity. Nichols (1989, p. 109) argues that entry into the typical general hospital involves adoption of a role whose central feature is *'required helplessness'*. Not surprisingly in the face of these experiences, clients generally welcome opportunities for decision-making and control, even when these cannot directly influence the course of illness itself. Individuals living with long-term physical, cognitive and emotional difficulties particularly need to exert choice over the decisions that will affect their future lives, yet their voice in such decision-making is often excluded.

Communications that support clients' decision-making and control are central to empowerment. The 'building blocks' of good communication that have already been described, such as active listening, providing information and inviting clients to contribute to the therapeutic encounter through open questions, all enhance clients' participation in decision-making and their ability to control outcomes. When clients feel fully part of the team and its decision-making processes, they are more motivated to take a committed role in the therapeutic process (Ley 1988).

There is some argument about how much specialist information clients require to help them in making difficult decisions. Some clients wish to receive (or to research for themselves) the scientific evidence about their treatment. Where clear evidence for the effectiveness of a treatment exists, knowledge of this would appear to motivate many clients to be optimistic about likely outcomes. However, therapists need to make more complex judgements about evidence in relation to other therapies and ways of living with illness and impairment. One client with arthritis may believe that Tai Chi helps to preserve his mobility. Should the therapist who cannot find any 'scientific' evidence, based on randomized controlled trials, to support the client's belief, nevertheless accept that for this man the practice of controlled, slow movements offers a valued sense of mastery over his body and illness? When the client feels able to promote his or her personal health, then emotional and physical well-being become much more attainable. Therapists require sensitivity to their clients' preferred strategies of maintaining control. Although clearly health-jeopardizing strategies should not be encouraged (such as excessive drinking of alcohol), therapists can do much to help clients preserve valued roles and activities. These offer a potent means of exercizing meaningful and satisfying control over life and identity.

Conscientization – raising awareness of disabling cultural forces

The traditional medical approach to treatment and rehabilitation still tends to individualize clients' problems, viewing the person's own efforts at learning and adaptation as primarily responsible for 'overcoming' disability. Disabled people are, therefore, often left to discover the social model of disability haphazardly, by themselves. Yet by moving to a position of viewing disability as both a personal and a public or political issue, the disabled person becomes empowered to confront the cultural stereotypes, discrimination, and environmental barriers that undermine quality of life and identity (Swain & Cameron 1999, Williams 2001). Consciousness raising has been seen as a legitimate aspect of health promotion, particularly by feminist therapists, and by some working in mental-health settings (Israeli & Santor 2000, Townsend et al. 2000). Along similar lines, Peters (1999) argues that positive identity can be derived through conscientization, the process of making more visible the implicit social and cultural values that oppress disabled people. Perhaps therapists could do more to promote discussion with clients about these wider forces. For example, a therapist who hears a client referring to herself as 'worthless' (or in other negative terms) during therapy may encourage some reflection on the language we draw from the wider culture that derides impairment and disability.

Of course, therapists should not pressurize clients into simply replacing any negative self-references with politically 'correct' language. Consciousness raising needs to go deeper, involving a sometimes lengthy process of addressing personal and social values, reinterpretation of priorities in life, and social activism. Clients who are initially very negative about their physical condition and social status as a disabled person can be better supported in 'rethinking' disability by contact with groups who are confronting similar challenges (as will be discussed further in Chapter 9). There is also a rich body of literature (political and autobiographical) written by disabled people, and some clients may be willing to read further to gain insights into others' experiences and their increasingly successful advocacy for equal rights. They may also appreciate knowing more about the Disability Discrimination Act, and their various entitlements. Therapists might also encourage greater awareness of the disabling forces that operate within the local rehabilitation and hospital environment, supporting clients in advocating for services that better respect their rights and needs.

Reflections

In your work with an elderly man who has had a stroke, you hear him say, 'I'm no good, I'm completely useless now'. Think about some ways in which you could encourage him to see himself more positively, whilst also offering empathy.

SELF-EXPRESSION THROUGH NARRATIVE AND ART

So far, the chapter has primarily focused on the day-to-day skills that therapists need to build effective working alliances with their clients. There are a number of further communication skills and strategies, although these are usually associated with specialist settings, and/or formal counselling.

Some users of services have a pressing need to make sense of their lives, and to move on. Refugees and asylum seekers, victims of torture, people who have acquired profound physical impairments, and people with extensive experience of institutional living, including some people with learning difficulties, may need to engage in life review processes in order to come to terms with events and impose some meaning or sense of order. Gaps may need to be remembered and completed through the repeated re-tellings of the life story. The stories also need to be *witnessed*. 'There is a role . . . for therapists, and other practitioners, in recognizing that everyone has a story to tell and in *listening* to that story. Being listened to may be the first step in the telling of the life story and the reclaiming of identity' (Atkinson 1999, p. 11). Atkinson has engaged in life review with people who were judged many years ago to need institutional care because of their learning difficulties. For many, contact with family and information about their early years had been lost, leaving large gaps in their autobiographies and, therefore, a sense of rootlessness. Life review was conducted through narrative, and through examining and collating the records of the person's life to be found in case notes, archives, public record offices and photographs. Participants found this to be a valuable experience.

Therapists need to be mindful that some people have endured such trauma that their experiences are essentially 'unspeakable'. They may find it emotionally safer to express distressing memories and feelings through non-verbal channels such as visual art (e.g. painting or pottery), or through body movement (including drama and dance). The creative arts can help people to deal with feelings in an 'oblique' or indirect way, rather than through direct and painful confrontation (Dekker 1996). Creative activities can also offer opportunities to celebrate achievement and identity. Artwork confirms the existence of the artist, as it leaves a tangible record. Over time, a series of paintings (or other pieces of artwork) can reveal change, growth and mastery to the client (Schaverian 1991). Art therapists differ in their use of verbal commentary. Whilst some seek to interpret the images that their clients create, others view the artistic process itself as the therapeutic, integrative experience (Pearson 1996). It is important for health professionals to be able to tolerate the pain and ambiguity of the visual image, otherwise they are likely to prevent clients from finishing the work that they need to do. One art therapist, interviewed about her work with people who have learning difficulties (Reynolds 1999b), described how a client had repeatedly covered her paper in black crayon. The activities organizer had simply removed the black crayon, without any reflection on the deeper meaning of the woman's actions. The art therapist expressed concern that this action prevented the client from engaging in a grieving process.

Looking again at the example of Ken Walker, possibly the use of art during occupational therapy or counselling would have provided him with the means to externalize and master the shadow that was so terrifying to him. It may have opened up a channel of two-way communication between himself and the therapist.

There are many ways of introducing art into therapy for the purposes of enabling emotional expression, integration of experience and life review (see Graham-Pole 2000 for practical examples). One means of life review involves drawing a trajectory or time-line, on which the person places the life events and people that have been of most significance. The person has the freedom to present the life trajectory in any way that seems appropriate and satisfying. A straight line, a meandering river, a tangle of knots or any other representation of a line that has a personal resonance may be used. Once the life trajectory has been drawn, and perhaps labelled, the person may engage in further reflection to gain deeper self-understanding from the image created. Modification of the image can provide a powerful way of initiating change.

Therapists need to be mindful that the more specialist communication and counselling strategies have powerful effects in terms of emotional disclosure and relationship building. Further training and clinical supervision are recommended before using the creative arts methods outlined here. There are other creative techniques, usually conducted in a group setting, which help clients communicate their stories and build positive identities, such as reminiscence therapy, story-making, collage, dance and drama. Groups offer many other opportunities for empowerment, and these will be considered in the next chapter.

Reflections

Use a large sheet of paper, preferably A2 in size. You can stick four pieces of A4 together to form a large rectangle, if necessary. Plain paper is preferable, but lined paper will do. Using whatever imagery you like, represent your life to date by drawing a time-line, or map. You might choose to represent transitions and turning points, as well as achievements and losses on the line/map. You may add notes and labels if you wish. In constructing your time-line, do not edit it with an audience in mind. You are creating this as a communication to yourself. Take your time and use whatever creative strategies you like to represent on the paper what is most important to you. When you have finished, take time to reflect on the experience. What does the finished visual piece suggest to you? For example, is your imagery bold or faint? Simple or complex? Neat or messy? How do you interpret this? (There is no 'correct' answer, and your own interpretations may change with your mood and other experiences.) On another day, would your life's 'blueprint' change? What difficulties in finding adequate self-expression did you experience along the way? What difference did it make to your self-expression that you were creating primarily a visual image, not a verbal narrative? If you have a trusted fellow student or colleague, you might share the process of life review and your discoveries from the exercise.

CARING FOR YOURSELF

Two-way communication enables partnership and empowerment, but it can be emotionally taxing for the therapist to remain attentive, open to feelings and responsive to the individual stories and needs of their many clients. You will need certain strategies to care for yourself, so that you can remain a strong and effective ally of your clients, and able to invest enough of yourself in your therapeutic relationships. The most appropriate strategies for self-care vary from one individual to another, but you might consider the suggestions below.

Be realistic

Be realistic about what can be achieved within each encounter. Organizational factors generally limit the amount of time that you can spend with patients/clients. You may come to feel anxious that you never have sufficient opportunity for giving *enough* control, information and emotional support to clients. Yet therapists who genuinely communicate client-centred values, and listen to their clients even in brief encounters, will almost inevitably provide a significantly therapeutic experience. It will help you to address any sense of inadequacy if you focus on what you are achieving over several sessions rather than in a single session (Stewart et al. 1995).

Maintain boundaries

Identify the limits of your responsibilities and try not to take home your worries about clients. Work on developing the discipline of turning your full attention from one client to the next client's legitimate needs as you go through the day (Higgs 1991).

Be reflective

Regularly analyze what has gone well and not so well in your therapeutic work and communications and learn from these. Make your reflections explicit through discussion or diary work. Actively process any uncomfortable feelings that are surfacing in association with your work with clients.

Be creative

Use a full range of health-promoting strategies to maintain your well-being, including physical and creative activity, and other pursuits that are meaningful to you.

Training

If you work in a clinical setting that seems to be taking a toll on your emotions, do seek further training and professional development in communication and counselling skills.

Clinical supervision

Set up and use clinical supervision. This should be a vital non-judgemental arena for exploring difficult experiences with clients, and barriers to partnership.

Use the team

Encourage a whole-team approach: resist being the sole confidante and bearer of clients' distress.

Support

Recruit support from outside the one-to-one relationship both for the client and for yourself. Help clients to become aware of and use their own resources and support networks.

Note the positive

Take note of positive experience and change. Allow yourself to hear positive feedback from clients about their progress and satisfaction.

CONCLUSION

This chapter has acknowledged the wider forces that inhibit two-way communication between individual therapists and clients, but has focused on the personal qualities, such as empathy, and the communication skills, such as active listening, that therapists need if they are to create partnership approaches to therapy and rehabilitation. Communication in group contexts will be addressed in the next chapter.

Acknowledgements: I am grateful to the students of occupational therapy and rehabilitation counselling at Brunel University who have shared their experiences of clinical practice with me. I have drawn on several of their narratives to formulate the fictitious case example incorporated into this chapter. I am also grateful to those who provided personal narratives in my recent project on women's strategies of living with MS.

Chapter 9

Enabling relationships in group contexts

Frances Reynolds

Groups can provide the most enabling – and the most inhibiting – of contexts in which to communicate. Whether participants' experiences within a group are positive or negative depends upon a wide range of factors including the skills of the facilitator/leader, the norms governing social interaction, and perceptions of emotional safety. A great variety of therapy/support groups are found in health- and social-service settings (Doel & Sawdon 1999). Indeed, occupational therapists regularly lead groups in both physical- and mental-health settings (Cole 1998, Finlay 1997). Physiotherapists also recognize that group treatment provides a practical and effective alternative to working with individual clients (Gelsomino et al. 2000). Speech and language therapists adopt some group approaches to therapy, and have also been instrumental in setting up a participatory organization for people with aphasia, called 'Connect' (http://www.ukconnect.org).

In addition to receiving professionally led group treatment, disabled people are also increasingly recognizing the mutual support of self-help groups (Habermann 1990). Although the notion of 'self-help' has been criticized as perpetuating social pressures on disabled people to regain 'normality' (Marks 1999), many participants reject this argument and report that such groups make an impressive contribution to their quality of life and well-being (McWilliam et al. 1996, Stuifbergen & Rogers 1997). Many other social groups that are found in the community, including those associated with religion, and adult education, also play an important role in enabling support and integration for people with long-term health problems. This can make a vital difference, particularly to the well-being of people who become socially isolated after the onset of an illness such as a stroke (Ouimet et al. 2001). Generally, a group provides 'a place where individuals can find their voices, individually or together, learn together and challenge together' (Doel & Sawdon 1999, p. 25).

Groups are particularly valued by people who feel disempowered, whether it is by disease itself, or by disabling social processes such as stigmatization and discrimination. Serious illness or impairment is all too often a lonely experience, and the person may feel powerless – especially in the early stages – to cope or look ahead with any confidence. It can also be a humourless place in which the person confronts the most serious issues of life and mortality. For people facing such stressful experiences, a group can provide much needed antidotes, such as autonomy, playfulness, camaraderie, flexibility and humour (McWilliam et al. 1996).

There is a great deal of evidence that social support makes a tremendous difference to the quality of life – and even to the physical health – of people facing long-term illness and/or other adversities. Whilst support is often provided by families and friends, not everyone enjoys a wide social network. Nor do family, or work colleagues, necessarily stay supportive in the long term (Lackner et al. 1994). Over time, they sometimes forget, become impatient or lose interest in the person's needs. Among people with mental-health problems, social relationships can be particularly limited or conflictual. People with speech and language problems are frequently excluded from 'mainstream' social activities. Specially convened groups for support, self-help and therapy can provide the experience of inclusion that may be lacking in everyday life.

This chapter will explore some of the processes in groups that promote enabling communications, and some of the common barriers that inhibit open and supportive exchange. Implications for therapists facilitating group-work will be highlighted. We will firstly examine different types of groups, including educational, therapeutic and self-help groups, to clarify their various purposes. We will consider why in certain circumstances, groups provide a more enabling therapeutic context for participants than one-to-one work with a therapist. Group dynamics are affected by the complex interplay among factors such as the facilitators' skills, members' own reasons for participating, processes of social perception and stereotyping, and group climate. Barriers to effective interaction will be considered mostly in the context of therapist-led groups, to assist in the development of your facilitation skills. However, many issues are relevant to understanding the dynamics of user-led groups, as well as teams of health professionals. Throughout the chapter, discussion will highlight some of the skills and attitudes that contribute to effective facilitation of groups.

There are many examples of successful therapeutic groups in books and research articles. Selected references will enable you to read further if you wish. There is insufficient space here to consider the variety of theoretical models that guide groupwork, but the references will help you to learn more about these. In particular, the readers who are interested in psychodynamic perspectives on groupwork are advised to consult Ringer (2002). Roberts (1995) also provides a good overview of the historical development of group psychotherapy.

Although this chapter focuses mainly on professionally led groups in which clients participate, some of the issues around enabling and inhibiting dynamics will also help you to understand why certain teams of health professionals pull together more successfully than others, creating more productive, satisfying working environments.

TYPES OF GROUPS IN HEALTH CONTEXTS

Although groups have many different purposes and structures, a broad but useful distinction can be made between groups that are led by therapists/ health professionals, and those that are led by clients. For convenience, we will include in the second category individuals attending self-help groups for whom the designation as 'client' or 'user of therapy services' is not really appropriate. Participants in self-help groups are not 'patients' as such, but individuals living in the community who are coping with long-term health and social problems using their own self-management strategies. Professionally facilitated and user-led/self-help groups raise rather different issues around power and empowerment.

A second major distinction can be made in regard to whether the primary purpose of a group is educational, supportive or therapeutic. In educational groups, the main aim is to exchange information and ideas – for example about the health condition, available services and so on – and to empower choice. Educational groups frequently provide information verbally, but experiential and practical exercises may also be included. Indeed, one group of people with enduring mental-health problems who participated in a community living skills group rated their practical learning about everyday tasks as more enjoyable and memorable than the verbal discussion (Brown et al. 2001). Physiotherapists tend to offer educational groups that focus on learning and practising physical exercise, and movement strategies (e.g. to protect the spine and prevent low back pain). In educational groups, a health professional usually has the prime responsibility to provide expert information. Nevertheless, the members themselves may also have expertise that they share.

Support groups offer camaraderie and opportunities to share stressful experiences and coping strategies, and to promote self-esteem. Some are more explicitly oriented towards empowerment and social change, for example working towards better employment opportunities, campaigning against illicit drug use, and advocating better recognition for carers (Nylund 2000). They may also have an educational function. Although some support groups are facilitated by health- and social-care professionals, they are frequently user-led.

In therapeutic and personal growth groups, the main purpose is to provide a context for safely exploring feelings, problems, and goals, for gaining insight, and for achieving behavioural, cognitive or lifestyle change. A range of health professionals lead such groups, including occupational therapists, nurses, art therapists and psychologists. Advanced groupwork requires facilitators to have specialist skills and training, and ongoing clinical supervision. As well as helping clients to achieve personal insight and confidence, therapy and growth groups may also enable participants to work collectively to challenge the stigma and oppressive practices that they encounter in daily life. Doel & Sawdon argue that:

Empowerment, in the sense of an increasing feeling of self-worth and a growing ability to feel and use power in constructive ways, should be an integral part of the members' experience of the group. (1999, p. 51)

In practice, the conceptual distinction between educational, supportive and therapeutic groups sometimes becomes blurred. In a recent interview that I carried out, a woman with multiple sclerosis (MS) described how she had gained a personal insight of considerable therapeutic significance from attending an educational meeting about MS. In the educational session, a specialist MS nurse provided information about the physiological processes that give rise to the fatigue that is so characteristic of this disease. The interviewee was relieved to discover that recent research into nerve conduction had demonstrated a 'valid' physical reason for fatigue. This information was therapeutic in helping the woman to challenge her long-standing fears that she might be judged as 'malingering', and to allay her nagging suspicion that her profound fatigue symbolized, in some way, a personal moral weakness – an unwillingness 'to try hard enough'. She also described gaining other therapeutic benefits from sharing experiences of fatigue with others in the group. She had learned that group members were facing similar problems in their everyday lives, and valued sharing coping strategies for this debilitating aspect of MS. In regard to classifying groups as educational, supportive or therapeutic, it must also be noted that the 'same' group can be experienced differently according to participants' needs and preferred styles of coping. For example, a recent study showed that men with prostate cancer tended to value attending a self-help group for the information that was exchanged among group members about the disease and available treatment options. In contrast, their wives tended to appreciate the group for the opportunity to disclose worries and receive emotional support from people with first-hand knowledge of the problems that they faced (Gray et al. 2000).

Groups can also be differentiated according to whether they are open or closed. Self-help and most educational/support groups tend to be 'open', accepting new members throughout the group's life. As a consequence, participants regularly experience the departures of some members, and the arrivals of new ones, and cope with repeated change in the group's dynamics. Some therapy groups are 'closed', that is, their membership remains the same throughout the group's existence. For example, if a closed group is scheduled to meet eight times, it will not accept new members after the first session. The closed option is selected when trust, emotional safety and confidentiality are absolutely vital to the therapeutic process.

Doel & Sawdon (1999) point out certain further distinctions among groups that affect their pattern of functioning. Some groups are adapted from pre-existing groups that already live or work together, for example in a residential setting or a community organization, whilst others are created afresh. In adapted groups, at least some of the group members know each other beforehand. This tends to create a greater risk of pre-formed alliances or cliques within the group, and the possibility of 'emotional baggage' being brought into the group from the other contexts in which the individuals meet.

However, such previously established relationships can be useful for speeding up the development of trust and the ability of the group to decide upon its preferred ways of working. Group dynamics are also affected by other factors, such as whether attendance at the group is voluntary or compulsory, whether the life of the group is open-ended or time-limited, and whether the group follows a tightly organized or loose programme. Whilst groups usually provide a highly interactive context, in some cases – such as a studio art group – members may primarily work in parallel, perhaps only interacting at the end of a session yet drawing comfort from the physical presence of others who share similar difficulties (McGraw 1999).

EXAMPLES OF GROUPWORK IN HEALTH AND SOCIAL CARE

Groups have been used widely by occupational therapists in the treatment and support of a wide variety of clients, including those with physical- and mental-health problems. Groupwork occurs in both in-patient and community-treatment settings. To give a few examples, occupational therapists have found groupwork particularly relevant in mental-health settings for assisting clients with anxiety (e.g. Prior 1998), and for supporting people with psychosis (e.g. Hyde 2001). Mothers of children with long-term impairments described an occupational therapy group programme as helpful for building further awareness of how to care for their children, and for regaining a positive self-image (Helitzer et al. 2002). Various group education programmes have been offered by occupational therapists such as energy conservation for people with MS (Mathiowitz et al. 2001). Physiotherapists have also recognized the value of groupwork, and not only for its potential to offer cost-effective treatment (Demain et al. 2001, Gelsomino et al. 2000). A wide range of articles report that physiotherapy group treatments in both in-patient and primary-care settings increase clients' knowledge, motivation and social support – for example in the context of managing chronic back pain (Penttinen et al. 2002), incontinence (Demain et al. 2001), spinal-cord injury and stroke (Gelsomino et al. 2000). Taskinen (1999) reported that an exercise group for people with hemiplegia, meeting over 24 sessions, not only increased fitness; participants experienced the group as motivating and rewarding, enhancing their quality of life. For people with communication difficulties, therapy groups offer a naturalistic opportunity to practise conversational skills with others who understand the difficulties and frustrations that can occur. Such group therapy has been shown to have beneficial outcomes (Elman & Bernstein-Ellis 1999).

Many other health- and social-care professionals facilitate client groups including nurses, social workers, youth workers, group psychoanalysts, psychologists and creative arts therapists. Selected examples include groups to support people with cancer (Minar 1999, Predeger 1996, Serline et al. 2000); HIV/AIDS (Getzel & Mahoney 1989, Piccarillo 1999); terminal illness (Firth 2000); schizophrenia (Mason 2000); depression, loss and bereavement (Riley 2001, Rishty 2000); eating disorders (Ball & Norman 2000, Doktor 1996); and learning disabilities (James 1996, Read et al. 2000). Groupwork has also been shown to help individuals who have suffered traumatic experiences, such as sexual abuse (Nosko & Breton 1997–8) or the suicide of loved ones (Constantino & Bricker 1996). Carers can also benefit from learning skills and sharing experiences in a group context (e.g. as Booth & Swabey (1999) have shown with carers of people who have aphasia).

Self-help groups have partly evolved in response to patients' dissatisfaction with the quality of information and advice that is made available by biomedically oriented health practitioners. Equally importantly, self-help groups enable participants to offer each other mutual support through sharing experiences, strategies, and practical help on an equal basis. However, it is to be noted that individuals with more severe impairment and fewer resources may find it difficult to access such groups, as Code et al. (2001) has shown in their profiling of self-help groups for people with aphasia. Nevertheless, the internet has brought into being many 'virtual' self-help groups, enabling people to share experiences without the physical barriers of access, distance and transport that would have to be overcome if they were meeting face-to-face. For example, a virtual self-help group called Jooly's Joint, has been created by Julie Howell, for people with MS (http://www.mswebpals.org). It has received design awards and positive feedback from users. For example, one posting states 'The caring here comes to you like a big snuggly blanket'. Such 'virtual' support groups may be particularly welcomed by people with severe mobility problems.

In terms of 'typical' group activities, many educational and self-help groups aim to provide a regular forum for verbal exchange of information and discussion. Therapy groups generally participate in a much wider variety of interactional strategies, including creative activities. Examples include role play, life review, guided fantasy, and creative artwork, including art, music and drama. Doel & Sawdon (1999) suggest that different media offer distinctive possibilities for therapeutic insight and interaction, and they describe visual techniques, such as art, collage and flip-charting, movement techniques, such as group sculpts, mime and role play, and verbal techniques, such as group story-making and reminiscence. By changing the medium of expression, a greater variety of emotional issues may become accessible, and open to exploration within the group. Furthermore, with diverse interactive techniques, the group dynamics run less risk of becoming predictable and 'fossilized'. However, it is important not to introduce interactive 'techniques' into the group simply for variety, without a deep consideration of their therapeutic purpose.

Occupational therapists and arts therapists make use of a wide range of creative tasks and techniques to promote interaction in groups. Why are creative activities considered to be so enabling? The primary purpose of focusing on creative artwork in groups is to aid members to express their deeper feeling obliquely, with less risk of painful confrontation or shameful verbal disclosure (Riley 2001). The creative focus helps to assure emotional safety. Some people regard their experiences as so painful that they are essentially 'unspeakable'. In such cases, any attempt by the facilitator to elicit explicit verbalization would most likely arouse defences and avoidance strategies. Creative artwork in groups enables members to share their experiences non-verbally, to make tentative connections with each other at a pace that they can control, and to gain validation and support. Use of imagery and metaphor may permit safer exploration of personal issues. Creative activities are also interesting, sustaining attention and promoting a meaningful focus for interaction, even for individuals struggling with cognitive impairments. For example, Riley (2001) described group artwork and collage with older people with dementia and physical frailty. She described how the group worked together over a number of sessions to co-construct a village scene embodying the theme of community. The group task was partially led by the residents themselves, and they participated to the degree that their cognitive and physical skills allowed, with even 'minor' contributions having evident importance in the final product. The task helped members to focus on their strengths, and to access precious memories. Rishty (2000) has taken a similar approach to reminiscence groupwork with older adults. Through structured creative activity, participants in both cases were able to experience a sense of inclusion and valuing, even when their capacity to interact in more usual, less structured, social contexts was severely impaired. Riley (2001) suggests that the finished collage provided a visible record of the group's achievement, enabling all participants to feel pride in the group and self-esteem. Clearly the facilitators' skills for weaving together the disparate contributions of group members and communicating unconditional acceptance were vital to the group process, as in all forms of groupwork.

You need to be mindful that advanced therapeutic groupwork techniques require further training and supervision. With all forms of communication that assist people to address deeply painful issues (and possibly to dismantle long-standing psychological defences) it is important that the facilitator has sufficient skill to maintain the emotional safety of all participants, including him/herself. Psychodynamic theory is often used by facilitators of psychotherapeutic groups to guide and interpret the group dynamics. Further theoretical insights into psychodynamic group therapy are offered by Ringer (2002).

IN WHAT WAYS MAY GROUPS OFFER MORE OPPORTUNITIES FOR EMPOWERMENT THAN ONE-TO-ONE COMMUNICATIONS?

Groups – when they function well – appear to offer more opportunities for empowerment than one-to-one communications between therapist and client.

The interviewee (in the Reflections exercise box below) seems to value the permission within the group to drop façades and receive empathy from other centre users who share the disease and the problems that it creates for daily life. Many people with serious illness, such as cancer, have noted difficulties with honest self-presentation and the burden of pretence. They often feel an obligation to be strong and uncomplaining with family and friends in order not to increase their worries (Predeger 1996). The interviewee also seems to welcome the opportunity to be open and honest about the difficulties posed

Reflections

The following statement was provided by a young woman with MS about some of her experiences of attending an MS Therapy Centre (a charitable centre that provides both professional services and self-help groups). Examine her account in which she describes interacting with other centre members. What do you consider is potentially therapeutic about her experiences in this particular self-help group?

> Since I have had MS, I have met a load of really brilliant people. People with a lot of courage and a lot of guts and humour. And also people who are very genuine. I go to the MS centre once a week and sometimes that is what psychologically keeps me going during the week, because we have such a good laugh there. We come in and we'll say, 'You look blooming awful!' And then we'll all laugh because we all look awful! And we can just be ourselves. Sometimes you have to get into context the idea of you having a disability but still being a person. And it is very difficult when other people see you as someone with a disability and maybe not as a person. You've got to have some kind of self-image and it is very difficult because it keeps shifting. You have to keep an intrinsic self-image of self-worth inside you, otherwise you would fall apart. And I think that is the process really.

by illness (such as its effects on mobility and appearance). This view resonates with the findings of various studies. In everyday life, many people with substantial health problems sense that others are embarrassed by their illness. Some also fear that disclosure will lead to their illness becoming an all-defining 'master status' in the eyes of others (Mathieson & Stam 1995). For the interviewee, the open acceptance of others, including their use of teasing and humour, promotes inclusion and confirms her positive identity and status as a person with equal worth. Positive self-worth is not always validated in 'mainstream', more disabling environments. Furthermore, in the group setting, the interviewee is also active in offering support and affirmation to others, and perhaps derives some satisfaction from doing so. Clearly these various experiences, gained from interacting with people who have direct experience of the illness and its challenges, cannot be readily obtained in one-to-one work with a therapist.

Groupwork limits the dependence of group members on the therapist, compared with one-to-one therapy. Through group interaction and joint action on projects, members may accomplish more than they could alone, thereby gaining power and self-esteem. A sense of agency is particularly likely when the group members take over the running of the group themselves.

We can summarise some of the enabling experiences that commonly occur within group contexts, as follows:

- empathy, acceptance and validation
- expert advice and information
- emotional and practical support
- challenge and a stimulus for change
- opportunities to take on valued roles
- social facilitation effects and role modelling
- developing social skills and insights
- transcendence – moving beyond self
- consciousness-raising and political activism.

Empathy, acceptance and validation

Groups of individuals who share similar social and physical difficulties can provide a unique degree of empathy and acceptance, helping people to feel validated and understood, to feel pride rather than shame, and to clarify their own experiences and goals:

> What the patient needs is contact, to be able to touch others, to voice concerns openly, to be reminded that he or she is not only 'apart from' but is also 'a part of' others. (Yalom 1985, p. 23)

Validation may be particularly prized by people who feel isolated or judged negatively by wider society. For example, mothers of children with physical impairments reported finding strength and resilience through the respect and acceptance gained in an occupational therapy group (Helitzer et al. 2002). Individuals used to being labelled and dismissed as 'psychotic', found validation as 'complete' persons within a group for people with mental-health problems (Hyde 2001). Riley (2001) discusses her experiences conducting an art group for children who were recovering from severe burns. She emphasized that the children were very keen to tell their stories among peers who really understood their experiences, and who would accept them (and their scars) without judgement.

Expert advice and information

Groups of people who share similar health problems and issues around disability can assist each other in finding satisfactory ways of living with illness and impairment, through sharing their expertise – both in the form of information, and also their 'tried and tested' coping strategies. Stuifbergen & Rogers quoted an interviewee with MS saying that others with MS have:

> ... taken away a lot of the fear and have told me over and over ... 'You can still have this quality and do everything you always wanted to do, you just have to make adjustments for it' [the illness]. (1997, p. 13)

On some issues, group members with direct experience of a health or social problem are likely to provide more credible advice and information than a therapist who views the problem from an 'outsider' perspective. Gray et al. quote a participant whose husband had prostate cancer:

> ... he needed to go to the support group to talk to people about some of the physical ramifications of the operation. (2000, p. 536)

Clearly the official medical account of what to expect post-operatively was not sufficient.

Wilson (1999) acknowledges the growing expertise of people living with chronic illness, especially with the growth of access to the internet, which offers so many opportunities for researching information. Group members can gain considerable empowerment from pooling their knowledge and other resources.

Emotional and practical support

People with certain illness, such as cancer, frequently limit whom they tell about their diagnosis and worries (Gray et al. 2000). They feel obligated to put others' needs before their own in both family and work contexts, leaving themselves with little social support. Reflecting on an art therapy group for women with breast cancer, Minar writes:

> Being involved in an art therapy group gave the patients a way to express all of their complex feelings in an accepting environment where they did not have to put on a happy face to make those around them feel comfortable. (1999, p. 239)

Groups can provide not only emotional, but also practical support, which makes a significant difference to people's well-being. Support can provide the vital aid for personal adjustment as well as collective political action (Bender & Ewashen 2000). Many participants regard their education and therapy groups as a comfort and companion in their journey through illness. For example, one woman with breast cancer wrote:

> I see this group as a safe harbor from the storm of life around me. It is comforting to be among and gather strength from all of you. (Predeger 1996, p. 54)

For others, the group provides more than emotional nurturance. The support of other members can increase the person's confidence to engage in therapy, thereby maximizing the effectiveness of the treatment programme. For example, in an evaluation of back-care groups, Penttinen et al. (2002) compared outcomes in nine back-care groups who received 'normal' physio-therapy treatment with nine groups in which members were encouraged to interact socially and provide mutual support, in addition to practising their exercises. Longitudinal follow-up evaluations showed that quality of life and functional gains were greater in the treatment-with-social-support groups. Clearly, groups can provide far more mutual support among members, than the therapist working alone can offer.

As a further advantage of groupwork, relationships forged within educational and self-help groups may also extend into the person's life outside the group. However, it must be noted that generalization of group relationships into outside friendships may not be encouraged in psychotherapeutic groups, in order to maintain the confidentiality and trust of all group members.

Groups provide a challenge and a stimulus for change

Because of the different perspectives that are usually present among groups of individuals, communications in a group context can help to challenge members' negative assumptions about themselves, illness and disability, and may encourage positive attitude and behavioural change (e.g. self-advocacy). Through sharing perspectives, members can test the reality of their own beliefs and assumptions, a process that is of particular value for individuals coping with psychotic symptoms (Hyde 2001). However, certain dynamics can make a challenge by other group members appear threatening rather than enabling. Facilitators of groups need skills to manage such encounters. Such issues will be considered later.

Opportunities to take on valued roles

Groups often provide opportunities for members to take on new roles, helping to demonstrate each person's worth, and offering the experience of inclusion or partnership, regardless of degree of impairment or ill-health. This may be a particularly empowering experience for clients with severe physical or mental health problems who are often largely excluded from 'normal' roles in mainstream society. Those who have retired on grounds of ill-health or impairment may also enjoy using previously developed skills in the service of the group. For example, they may use previously acquired business skills to manage the agenda of a self-help group, to organize its paperwork, or to raise funds. Groups are microcosms of wider social situations (Yalom 1985), so group members who learn skills and confidence within a group may be able to transfer this learning into everyday life. Through harnessing the resources of many different members, the group is likely to be able to accommodate the impairments of specific individuals. The group's work can then provide a stimulus and sense of achievement that would be difficult for individual members to gain in isolation. For example, Crimmens (1998) reports on a storymaking drama group for people with dementia. Each member was enabled to participate in terms of his or her strengths and abilities. Even withdrawn members took on a valued role as audience to the unfolding drama. Such experiences seemed to counter the confusion and passivity that the participants more usually experienced in the everyday world of the nursing home. Furthermore, the author emphasizes that by encouraging members in group interaction to draw on their individual strengths (such as their vivid memories of their past lives, and their, sometimes, detailed knowledge of the historical events that they had directly witnessed), staff (and fellow residents) were better able to relate to the person rather than the dementia.

The group setting – with appropriate facilitation – can provide opportunities for group members to try out new and unfamiliar roles. In so doing, the person, and other group members, including staff, may recognize traits and capabilities in the individual that had previously been overlooked. For example, James (1996, p. 25) writes of a group activity for people with learning difficulties in which the group members took turns in leading or being blindfolded. The sister of one member had always taken on the role as carer to her disabled brother. She was amazed by the experience of being blindfolded and then being led by him. He showed such care and understanding in guiding her and helping her to explore the environment by touch. After the blindfolds were removed the group formed again to discuss the experience. James reports that the sister 'said that something rather amazing had happened which had opened up a whole new dimension to her relationship with her brother. She had met him in an entirely new and different light . . . ' Nosko & Breton (1997–8, p. 57) also argue that it is important for facilitators to 'promote a group context and programme in which [participants] can demonstrate and share their specific strengths', helping them to move beyond the conventional labels and stereotypes that may have limited their actions and self-image in the past.

Social facilitation and role modelling

If attitudes of group members are favourable to the task in hand, the presence of other group members will tend to maximize individual effort and motivation. This effect has been termed 'social facilitation'. Research over many years has shown that individuals tend to work harder and perform better in front of a group of peers, particularly those whose judgement they respect (Aiello & Douthitt 2001). This additional motivation may be particularly valuable in the physiotherapy setting (Gelsomino et al. 2000). For example, the social facilitation effect can encourage people to gain the confidence to try new exercises and safer ways of moving and lifting. With increased motivation and commitment to learning from the group, individuals may gain much more from therapy, leading to successful learning and greater satisfaction with the programme. Role modelling also regularly occurs during group interaction, with participants imitating the behaviour not only of the therapist, but also other group members. This process can also facilitate the acquisition of skills, and self-confidence, promoting achievement.

Developing social skills and insights

Groups have a potential for replaying family dynamics, therefore helping members to gain insight into their long-standing conflicts and habitual responses to others. These issues form a particular focus in some therapy and personal growth groups. However, just as siblings squabble for attention, so too can group members (Doel & Sawdon 1999). This can be detrimental to the group's functioning unless managed skilfully by the group facilitator, in a way that encourages reflection and insight among all participants. Some groups, particularly for people with enduring mental-health problems or learning difficulties, enable the practice of social skills during structured tasks that are designed to minimize anxiety and failure. Again, the value of the group is that it presents a microcosm of the social world. Increased confidence and interactive skills within the safe context of the group is thought likely to transfer into other settings, assisting in integration and quality of life. In some groups, as members gain the confidence to direct the process themselves, the therapist gradually withdraws and enables group members to take over the running of the group (Steiner 1992).

Transcendence – moving beyond self

Groups offer the opportunity for transcendence – to move beyond the narrow confines of self and illness, and to embrace a wider purpose or find deeper meaning. This may be one motive for people joining self-help groups. Commitment to a group project, such as a community art project, helps people to feel less isolated or overwhelmed by illness. The group may be able – through pooling their ideas and skills – to create an artistic product that the individuals working alone could never have envisaged. Individuals can also experience transcendence through banding together to create organizations that bring lasting benefits to others. For example, people with MS have set up a number of charitable therapy centres. Fund-raising and other activities require much group effort and commitment, but participants achieve much satisfaction from their achievements in bringing valuable resources to people who would otherwise receive relatively little therapeutic help. Helping others increases self-efficacy and self-esteem (Schwartz & Sendor 1999).

Consciousness–raising and political activism

Some group facilitators explicitly value groupwork as a stimulus to social action. For example, Nosko & Breton argue, in connection with their work with abused women, that the support group helps 'the women to identify the common social, political, economic and cultural contexts of their situations' (1997–8, p. 56). Groups increase the power of individuals to gain a wider social perspective on their individual problems, and to create pressure for social change. For example, a group of disabled people is likely to be a more formidable force for change (e.g. in advocating for more appropriate local services, access and other resources) than single individuals.

WHAT ARE THE COMMON BARRIERS TO ENABLING COMMUNICATIONS IN A GROUP CONTEXT?

Whilst groups can offer many enabling experiences, there are in practice many potential barriers to effective interaction.

Reflections

Before reading on, please reflect on (a) a group in which you have felt very comfortable to learn, interact and to express yourself, and (b) a group in which you felt very uncomfortable and inhibited. Think carefully about the factors that gave rise to these positive and negative experiences and, if possible, share your ideas with a colleague to see if there are any common patterns.

Groups can be productive or unproductive, enabling or disabling, depending upon a number of factors. It is difficult to provide an exhaustive list as each group – like each individual participating in a group – is unique. Nevertheless, the following appear to be common barriers to effective groupwork.

- Lack of ground-rules (e.g. confidentiality, permission to join in and disclose personal experience at one's own pace) will jeopardize members' feelings of security/safety.
- Insufficient attention and time given to building a supportive group climate.
- Over-emphasis on the group's task or product rather than its interactional processes or emotional climate. In creative arts groups, this orientation signals that artistic ability is valued over and above participation in the group. Groups that are very task-oriented are frequently unsupportive and careless with members' needs and vulnerabilities, and they risk later fragmentation (Johnson & Johnson 2002).
- An over-directive, over-interpretative or laissez-faire facilitator. These behaviours tend to increase the passivity, dependence or anxiety of group members.
- An inexperienced facilitator who feels a need to 'rescue' members, short-circuiting the possibility of genuine emotional expression or the building of trust.
- Domination by specific members' needs, or cliques.
- Involuntary membership.
- Poor resources/unsuitable environment.
- A clumsy closure to the group.
- Members having insufficient power, opportunity or resources to transfer therapeutic gains made within the group into their own environment.

Reflections

Consider the following case study, and put forward some suggestions for how the facilitators might have increased the acceptability and usefulness of the group.

CASE EXAMPLE: WHERE DID THE FACILITATORS GO WRONG?

An occupational therapist, physiotherapist, speech and language therapist, nutritionist and specialist MS nurse planned a group for people with MS living in the community. They decided to offer an educational group programme running over 7 weeks, with a 2-hour meeting each week. Each professional decided to take the lead in providing information on their specialist areas. The following topics were delivered:

1. What is MS?
2. New research into effective treatments for MS.
3. Fatigue management.
4. Dealing with incontinence, speech and memory problems.
5. Keeping fit: the importance of diet and exercise.
6. Discrimination issues: disablism, racism, and disempowerment.
7. Thinking positively.

A student therapist who attended the sessions thought that they were very well prepared and very informative. However, the health professionals were surprised to find that attendance declined markedly over the 7 weeks, and that the evaluation of the programme by those attending was very mixed. Whilst some group members had found certain aspects of the information very useful, they also made some sharp criticisms. Many of those attending thought that the information was mainly relevant to people newly diagnosed with MS. A large number already knew about the need for exercise and a healthy diet, but found it difficult – either because of mobility problems or financial difficulties – to put their knowledge into practice. The practical barriers that the group members experienced in acting upon advice had not been discussed in depth, nor had any useful strategies been planned during the group session. Some found the presentation patronizing, and said that the professionals seemed discomforted and defensive when one or two of those attending questioned whether the findings being presented had now been superseded by new research. Some also questioned whether people without personal experience of illness and disability could really tell disabled people how to think positively about their situation.

There was little opportunity to share experiences, ideas and strategies with others who were attending. Even the tea break was too short for meaningful interaction. Many had attended specifically in order to meet others who shared similar difficulties. Because interaction had been so limited, they had not received the opportunity to forge social networks. Members perceived that the very limited group discussion that took place had been dominated by two individuals. One man in the audience regularly spoke up to emphasize his belief that people with MS needed to pray and maintain their religious faith. The other dominant person referred repeatedly to her need for a reliable carer. The domination of the already limited discussion by two group members alienated many others.

Those attending lived in a rural part of the South of England and had little day-to-day acquaintance with the problems faced by people of ethnic minorities. They, therefore, reported in their feedback that the connections being made between social discrimination against disabled people and ethnic minorities were unconvincing and irrelevant to their experience. They stated that they would have preferred to have focused upon their own personal experiences of stigma and discrimination. They would also have liked to have formulated some strategies within the group to counter discrimination at the local level (for example, in lobbying a local company for a more accessible bus service).

This is a classic case of a group being used simply as an audience for information-giving by professionals who were well intentioned, but who had limited group facilitation skills. They had focused on delivering their own expertise but had ignored the group process, and the potential resources of each group member. As often happens, the negative feedback then splintered the team of health professionals, who started to blame each other for the relative failure of the group programme. It also fuelled their pre-existing stereotypes of people with MS being 'angry' and 'difficult'. The group's failure undermined the potential of the professional team to work co-operatively together in the future.

> ## Reflections
>
> What basic facilitation skills and strategies would have greatly improved the potential of the group to be educational, supportive and enabling? Consider your own ideas before moving on.

Even within the confines of quite a structured, educational group programme, the programme facilitators could have enhanced group functioning by following at least some of the below-mentioned recommendations. These suggestions may be applied in most educational and supportive group programmes.

When considering setting up a community group, a more appropriate programme can be developed from consultation with a small group of local people to discover what information would be useful, and what support needs they might have. In addition to planning the broad objectives of the group, the weekly programme can be drawn up in conjunction with people who have direct experience of the disabling health/social problem to maximize its relevance. In groups receiving a formal presentation of information, some speakers with direct experience of illness may be invited to address the group, to not only provide information, but also facilitate open discussion about the more personal, distressing aspects of illness, and to share personal coping strategies.

Facilitators need to avoid assuming that the audience knows nothing about the topics in question. Group members may wish to share information that they have researched, to share skills for researching information, and to discuss the practicalities (e.g. of diet, or exercise) in a personal sense (not just to receive information). Participants may wish to modify the agenda. They may wish to consider selected issues and search out information and ideas over the next week. By bringing back such material, the group gains some personal ownership over the programme and engages in active learning.

Considerable attention to the group process is required: ice breakers may be included at the start of the programme to help those attending to feel comfortable with each other and to begin the process of meaningful exchange. Structured discussion activities, especially at the beginning of a professionally led group can alleviate members' anxiety about participating in a new social context (Riley 2001).

Facilitators need to have a flexible repertoire of group activities to draw upon in structured group programmes, so that choice can be made according to the group's expressed needs, rather than simply imposing activities autocratically on the group. Ground rules with the group may need to be established regarding confidentiality, if sensitive issues are likely to be disclosed by group members. Ground rules may also cover the need for turn-taking, rather than domination of the conversation by single individuals, and respect for each others' contributions.

Facilitators need to model empathic, respectful behaviour. Listening skills and emotional sensitivity are as important when leading a group as when working with individual clients.

If it seems appropriate to those attending, the group may be broken into subgroups, each with a different agenda. Sometimes different groups for individuals with different needs may be required. Those who are newly diagnosed or those more experienced in the health condition (or older or younger, male or female) may have quite different perspectives. For example, Mason (2000b) discusses how people struggling with a first episode of schizophrenia are more expressive of their anxieties with others who are in the same situation. Fears about their long-term prospects, identity and capacity to cope may *increase* if they join a group of individuals who have enduring mental-health problems.

Facilitators need to encourage the formation of a genuine group by encouraging meaningful interaction among all members. As one strategy, the meeting could be punctuated with small group discussions and feedback, to increase the opportunity for everyone to speak. Leadership of discussion may be rotated. Members also need to be invited to offer suggestions for group activities and objectives. Some facilitators help group members to experience 'ownership' of the group by asking if they would decide upon a name for the group. For example, a group of older people with cognitive problems who worked on a collage together agreed on the name 'Young at heart, doing art' (Riley 2001).

Health professionals need reflective awareness of their own behaviour and personal comfort – for example, when communicating about sensitive or taboo topics, such as sexuality and continence. Open discussion within the group will be closed down if the health professionals themselves betray discomfort/embarrassment, or if they express affront when challenged.

Domination of the group by a single vociferous member, or small clique may require urgent attention if the group process is not to become distorted. One strategy is to invite regular small group (subgroup) discussions, which dilute and rotate the effects of the dominant member, and which encourage even quiet members to contribute. In some cases, overbearing group members need to be challenged directly. Doel & Sawdon (1999) point out that group members approve of the group leader exercizing power to manage conflict effectively.

An interactive tea/coffee break may provide another important opportunity for social interaction and the establishment of relationships that may persist afterwards if members so desire. Facilitators may invite reflective comment from group members about their perceptions of the group dynamics. If group members are encouraged to provide feedback on any emerging problem with the pattern of interaction, they may be able to find more effective ways of working together. Action taken by the whole group to manage disruptive or over-dominant members can be more effective than the attempts by the facilitator alone.

Productive group norms may be encouraged by facilitators who communicate the assumption that everyone has something of value to contribute and that participation, not passive listening, is going to be the norm for the group. If members perceive that passivity is the norm, they may find it progressively harder to alter their behaviour on subsequent occasions.

Facilitators may offer a variety of roles for different group members to encourage ownership of the group. For example, some group members may like to take on the responsibilities of taking minutes, publicizing the programme, seeking an external speaker, collecting some funds for tea and coffee, planning the next stage of the group, and so on. If regular small group discussion of topics is a feature of the programme, then rotation of the leadership of the small groups may be encouraged.

Some authors suggest keeping a 'here and now' ear so that issues that members are bringing in from the past or other contexts do not dominate the group's interaction (Riley 2001). Members may be invited to share how they are feeling, and coping in the present context, so that everyone can feel involved.

Facilitators need to understand how group dynamics evolve over time. For example, early meetings may be dominated by the process of establishing trust, and forming the norms that will underpin group behaviour. Only when trust has been established in the 'middle phase' of the group, is it likely that group members will feel able to disclose sensitive personal issues, or challenge the contributions of others appropriately.

Facilitators may wherever possible attempt to hand over power to the group, to decide on its own programme and to direct its own evolution. Riley argues that the 'group therapist unlocks the abilities of the group to be their own therapist. Fading in and out of leadership is a talent that must be developed' (2001).

The physical environment of the group requires attention, including access, seating arrangements that promote inclusion of all members, and so on. Facilitators need to be aware that some environments carry a stigma, and that groups (e.g. of people with enduring mental-health problems) may work far more effectively together in a neutral community venue than in a day hospital that communicates certain limited expectations about the group members, inadvertently maintaining their labels as 'patients'.

The closure of the group usually requires careful management. Even straightforward educational groups can mean a great deal to those attending. For example, people with hemiplegia attending an exercise group over 24 sessions saw the group as enhancing their quality of life (Taskinen 1999). When the group has ended, clients may miss the regular routine of going to the group, and the relationships that they have established there. Groups need to anticipate endings, and perhaps participants can be encouraged – if they wish to make further contact – to establish how to do this. It can also help the group to end positively if its achievements are celebrated, perhaps through a concrete memento, such as a photograph or other creative product. Members may be encouraged to set up a further self-help group, for longer-term support, if they so wish.

The above-mentioned suggestions will help you to lead educational, remedial and supportive groups in ways that are enabling rather than disabling. You need to note that facilitation skills for psychotherapy groups require much more attention to understanding the complexities of group dynamics, the roles that people are acting out in the group setting, and the emotional vulnerability of participants. To help maintain emotional safety, it is usual for pairs of therapists to co-facilitate psychotherapy groups. Much further training and supervision are required for the facilitators of such groups. For those of you who are taking your studies further, you are particularly recommended to read Doel & Sawdon (1999) and Johnson & Johnson (2002), as they explore group facilitation skills in considerable depth.

Chapter 10

Challenging walls of discrimination
John Swain

This chapter explores the possibilities for change through dismantling institutional discrimination and possible strategies of professional support for change. Emancipatory practice promotes awareness of and challenges to structural, environmental and attitudinal barriers to participation. This is an exploration of anti-discriminatory and anti-oppressive practice in challenging sexism, disablism, racism, classism, ageism, homophobia, and simultaneous oppression. Such challenges to discrimination build on a working alliance and effective communication to support inclusion and promote equality.

We look first at concepts and frameworks for thinking about emancipatory practice, with a particular emphasis on the principles of enabling relationships. From this basis we turn to practice, beginning with a narrative approach to empowerment and then examining emancipatory practice, particularly relating to disablism, racism and sexism.

WHAT IS EMANCIPATORY PRACTICE?

At this point we have reached the final component of turning principles of enabling relationships into practice and the task can feel particularly onerous. As Thompson points out, 'establishing a basis of equality and social justice in service provision is no easy matter' (2001, p. 162). In the face of different forms of discrimination and multiple discrimination, and also the vested power interests that obstruct change, there can be no simple formula solutions to developing therapy practice. Successful change will depend on collective commitment and action.

Nevertheless, as I hope will have been apparent in the book so far, the concerns we are pursuing under the flag of 'enabling relationships' have echoes and parallels in developing practice across a wide range of health- and social-care provision. This has meant that this book has been able to take an eclectic view of sources of ideas for developing enabling relationships. To give a specific example, Reimers & Treacher (1995) have put forward a set of principles for a 'user-friendly' style of counselling that offers a basis for anti-discriminatory practice in therapy. Their proposals, directed towards therapy practice, would include the following:

1. Therapy is essentially a human encounter between people who are human beings first, and therapist and client second. Failure to address power differentials, whatever their grounds, opens the door to abusive practice.
2. Therapists must accept that ethical issues are of primary importance in therapy practice. Ethical issues include the daily dilemmas of therapy with decisions about how best to give information, how much time to spend with people, how best to offer support, how to find some support for yourself or how to give your attention to someone you do not particularly like or respect.
3. An effective professional–client relationship is an alliance in which the interests, viewpoints and experiences from both standpoints are the material of negotiation.
4. Anti-discriminatory practice recognizes that difference of class, sexual orientation and other social divisions are part of the warp and weft of individual differences.
5. Clients' experiences of therapy and their satisfaction with therapy must form a crucial part of the evaluation of therapy practice.
6. Notions of anti-discriminatory practice necessitates recognition of the wider social environment in consideration of therapy practice and recognition too of the limitations of therapy.

It is useful at this point to return to the framework of principles in Chapter 6. Figure 6.1 depicts the framework for moving from theory to principles. Figure 10.1 below uses the same components to depict moving from principles to practice.

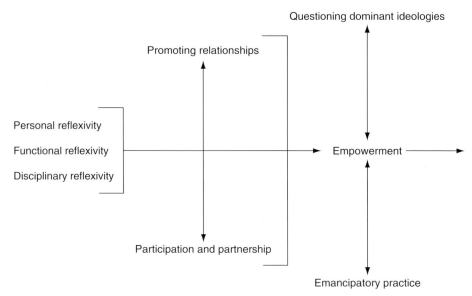

Fig. 10.1   From principles to practice in enabling relationships

It is not easy to depict human endeavours in a diagram and it can, indeed, be highly questionable if taken too literally. Nevertheless, we have reached the emancipatory practice components 'In practice' (questioning dominant ideologies, empowerment and emancipatory practice), although the diagram attempts to remind us that this is a cumulative and dynamic framework, and, thus, incorporates previous components (critical reflections and enabling relationships). As with all ostensibly progressive terminology, critical reflection remains central. Wilson & Beresford (2000), for instance, ask what constitutes anti-oppressive practice. They point out that, so far, clients and their organizations have had little significant involvement in the development of anti-oppressive theory and practice.

QUESTIONING DOMINANT IDEOLOGIES

The dominant ideologies relating to disability, as we have seen previously, are individualistic and tragedy models, including the medical model. The crucial development in questioning dominant ideologies, over at least the past 30 years, has been the establishment of the social model of disability. Through the social model, disability is conceived as something outside of the impaired individual. This model has supported disabled activists and their allies in challenging those aspects of the society that disable people with impairments. The first clear and principled statement of the social model is generally thought to be the statement by the Union of the Physically Impaired Against Segregation (UPIAS), a disabled people's organization, and took the form, centrally, of two definitions:

> *Impairment*: lacking part of or all of a limb, or having a defective limb, organ or mechanism of the body

> *Disability*: the disadvantage or restriction of activity caused by a contemporary social organisation which takes no, or little account of people who have physical impairments and thus excludes them from participation in the mainstream of social activities. Physical disability is therefore a particular form of social oppression. (Union of the Physically Impaired Against Segregation 1976, p. 14)

The social model has been significant in a number of ways. First, it stands in direct opposition to the dominant individualistic models of disability. In particular, the medical model insists that the difficulties faced by disabled people are a direct result of their individual impairments. The social model of disability recognizes the social origins of disability in a society organized and constructed by and for non-disabled people. The disadvantages or restrictions, often referred to as barriers, experienced by disabled people, permeate every aspect of the physical and social environment: attitudes, institutions, language and culture, organization and delivery of support services, and the power relations and structures of the disabling society (Oliver 1990, Swain et al. 1998).

Second, the social model of disability promotes the personal and political empowerment of disabled people. As Mercer & Barnes state, 'the medical approach concentrates on a set of discrete functional limitations requiring technical intervention and individual adjustment' (2000, p. 85). The social model engenders self-confidence and pride, rather than the guilt and shame associated with the individual tragedy model. The political implications of the social model, often explicitly stated, are to promote the collective struggle by disabled people for social change, equality, social justice and the rights of full participative citizenship.

Reflections

This exercise is adapted from Braye & Preston-Shoot (1995, p. 55). Think of the earliest time you remember being aware of someone who was disabled. What messages did you receive about your identity (as disabled or non-disabled) and other people's identity? What effect might this have had on your personal relationships and outlook, and on your work as a therapist? Ask yourself similar questions about class, race or ethnicity, and gender.

Think carefully about what disability means to you and try to define it. How is disability defined within the social model? Compare your definition of disability with the social model. Give examples from your experience of therapy practice that reflects an individual or medical model of disability. Give examples from your experience of therapy practice that reflect a social model of disability.

Questioning dominant racist ideologies involves: actively seeking awareness and understanding of our own racism and that of others; examining ways in which our attitudes, understandings and behaviour contribute to racism; and challenging and seeking to avoid cultural and racial stereotyping. Therapists wishing to challenge racism in their organizations need to begin along two lines suggested by Dominelli:

The first is that they subject their work to being monitored and evaluated by black people. The second is that they form anti-racist collectives with white people sharing their anti-racist objectives and develop ways of working together and supporting each other. (1997, p. 146)

Reflections

This exercise, to examine 'hidden' racism, is adapted from Dominelli (1997, pp. 86–89). It consists of a set of statements to be read and responded to in a discussion format by a group of white people. In discussion sessions, participants make spontaneous statements without them being judged. The

Continued

Reflections—continued

responses are then analyzed and assessed by the group to highlight any racist elements. I shall include a few of the statements here to give a flavour of the exercise and as provoking thought in terms of racism. The wording is changed where necessary to apply to therapists (rather than social workers as in the original). In what ways are the following statements racist?

1. Black clients come to the office with so many conflicting demands. What do they *really* want?
2. Racism is rare amongst therapists.
3. Other ethnic minority groups have settled in this country and improved themselves without 'positive discrimination'. Why shouldn't black people do likewise?
4. I'm not racist, I just think each ethnic group is different and should keep itself to itself. Black therapists should deal with black clients.
5. Every individual client should be judged on his or her merit.

Key aspects of racism identified, by Dominelli, in each of the above statements:

1. White people, from their sometimes assumed superior standpoints assume that black people do not know what they want. It is a way of trivializing their demands and struggles for racial justice.
2. Racism is defined as crude, irrational behaviour, thereby ignoring the significance of institutional and cultural racism on personal attitudes and action.
3. The person making the statement has failed to grasp the specific conditions surrounding black people's experiences of life in the UK. Society has changed and it is not the same as that of earlier groups of settlers.
4. Black people are held responsible for racism and for doing something about it. It suggests that there is no role for white people in deconstructing racism.
5. By looking at the situation in universal terms, the person is not recognizing the specificity of the black experience. It is structurally different from that of white people.

EMPOWERING STORIES

Notions of empowerment have been developed in practice in many different ways, some of which have been discussed in previous chapters. There is certainly no royal road for therapists in either empowering themselves or supporting the empowerment of others. One route explored by Ghaye & Lillyman is reflective conversation. They state:

> Reflective conversations which are empowering enable us to name, define and construct our own 'realities', to gain a greater sense of control over our professional lives and to develop a more authentic self. (2000, p. 64)

In their framework, reflective conversation is at the heart of the process of reflecting on practice. Reflective conversation between colleagues can be empowering for therapists. According to Ghaye & Lillyman (2000) the prime focus is on caring values, reflecting on your intentions in the therapy process – the ends you have in mind and the means for achieving them. There seem to be two associations with empowerment for clients:

1. Reflective conversations prioritize the meaning and value of the clients' viewpoint- what they bring to therapy, the meaning of therapy for clients and their evaluation of therapy in relation to their lives.
2. Critical reflection is creative in terms of support for clients in control over decision-making within the therapy process.

I shall concentrate next on an approach that builds on discussions in previous chapters: narrative. Narratives, or stories, provide a basis for empowerment as ways in which we make sense of ourselves and our lives, and frameworks for interpreting experience. How, then, might clients' narratives be incorporated into therapy practice, and how might this be empowering? Atkinson has argued that physiotherapy practice, by its nature, can provide a favourable milieu for narrative, and her argument can easily be extended to other forms of therapy:

> Therapists are well placed, through their work and in their relationships with clients, to play an active part in the telling of stories. This starts with recognizing that everyone has a personal past, and acknowledging and respecting that past. It goes further: it means listening to the life story when it is told; helping where possible, with the telling and the researching of that story; and recording the present sensitively, so that today's stories are recorded for the future in ways that people themselves approve. (1999, p. 21)

A narrative approach focuses on the stories that participants tell about their experiences. These stories can give therapists insight into motives, expectations, aims and convictions of the clients involved: 'A narrative can make us understand how people give meaning to a concrete situation and why they respond to it through a specific action. Narratives are not just descriptions of feelings and actions; they present these feelings and actions as part of a practice' (Widdershoven & Smits 1996, pp. 285–286). Narratives, for instance, have the power to illuminate experiences of illness and healing. They give meaning to illness, accident or impairment, the place of therapy within the unfolding story of responses to treatment, and re-telling of life history in the face of illness or impairment. McLeod suggests that:

> With non-professional, lay people, the form of understanding of account-ing for illness that is most often employed is the *story*. People tell stories about their health and illness. The sense of 'what made me unwell', 'how I feel today' or 'how I got better' is communicated to others through stories . . . People who are ill are often in a period of transition, struggling

to make the link between their pre-illness life-narrative and the story of who they are now. Achieving a coherent narrative can help give the person a sense of control and mastery over his or her condition, and can facilitate the process of establishing a viable role within their social group. Telling the story is a way of being known. . . . Allowing space for telling the story, and creating opportunities for the experience of being heard and understood, are part of effective health care. (1998b, pp. 51, 62–63)

Mattingly developed similar ideas in her work:

Life histories tend to emphasize the need for persons to find coherence and continuity in their lives . . . and telling a life story becomes one device by which persons try to interpret disruptive illnesses in life context . . . (1998, p. 13)

Through narrative, therapists come into contact with participants as people engaged in the process of interpreting themselves. Writing of her experiences using a life story approach in health-care research, Smith states:

Participants were seen to develop new insights into their personal experiences, family relationships, and social world understandings. They declared stronger feelings of self-value and personal rights; expressed increased confidence in the validity of their own perceptions; experienced greater integration of past events into their present sense of self; and presented an overall more centered, grounded, and self-cohering demeanor. (2000, p. 19)

Two key ideas in this type of narrative therapy are *deconstructing* the dominant narrative and *externalizing* the problem. The notion of deconstruction stems from the idea that people live their lives within the dominant narratives or knowledges of their culture and family, such as the individual medical and tragedy models of disability. This dominant narrative can conflict with personal experience (for instance, of the barriers facing people with impairments in a disabling society) and be in itself oppressive. Dominant cultural stories tend to concentrate on the norm or average behaviour in any particular situation and the norm becomes the desirable: normality. People who do not fit the norm are storied as 'abnormal' – the present-day equivalent of 'freaks' (Milner 2001). Practising narrative approaches involves challenging dominant cultural stories about problems. Listening to narratives can involve actively deconstructing the dominant narrative:

. . . the narrative therapist looks for hidden meanings, spaces or gaps, and evidence of conflicting stories. We call this process of listening for what is not said . . . (Drewery & Winslade 1997, p. 43)

As McLeod (1998a) explains, the process of externalizing the problem involves the client separating him or herself from the problem. Separating the person from the problem relieves the pressures of blame, defensiveness and perceived failure, and allows the person and his or her family to have a different relationship with 'the problem' – one in which resources are brought to bear on the social world rather than the person (Milner 2001). Furthermore, 'the device of externalization helps to reverse the trend in psychology toward seeking more and more deficits in human character and encouraging clients to relate to themselves as deficient human beings' (Drewery & Winslade 1997, p. 45). Thus the process of 'changing narratives' can be seen as part of the process of 'changing power relations'.

The notions of both deconstruction and externalizing the problem require therapists to access non-dominant or, what Thompson (1998) calls, countervailing ideologies, such as the social model of disability. This has been recognized, for instance, by Donati & Ward who take a critical stance to both the

---

Reflections

This is a shared narrative exercise, to explore narrative in the context of therapy. It involves both you and a client telling your stories of therapy. The following is a suggested format for the exercise, although you should adapt the steps to suit your particular situation.

1. You need to select a client with whom to undertake this exercise. This should be a client with whom a course of treatment is complete or with whom you have worked for some time.
2. Ethical considerations will be important from the outset, including of course informed consent and confidentiality.
3. It will be important to discuss the exercise with the client before listening to each others' stories. This should include ideas about what might be covered in the stories. As mentioned above, it is useful to listen for different possibilities within the story – uncertainties, possibilities for different interpretations and inherent contradictions. It is also useful to listen for changing directions in the story, points at which thinking changed – points of 'enlightenment'. You will need to discuss, too, the practicalities of the exercise, include method of recording the stories. This is best done by audio recording.
4. Getting into the exercise, first the client narrates his or her experience of therapy. Your role is to enable the client to tell his or her story. This involves a 'not-knowing' stance in relation to the client. The story you know is your story: the client is the expert on his or her story. It is crucial that you follow the client's lead, although listen in terms of the agenda agreed in your preliminary discussion.
5. Roles are then reversed: the client supports the therapist in telling his or her story. This should be conducted in a similar way to the first part of the exercise.
6. The final step is to share and discuss both stories: listening to the taped stories and exploring similarities and differences between the two stories.

medical model and educational approach in their work as occupational therapists and state:

> As a result of disability rights and independent living movements, the traditional view of disability has been redefined as one that locates the barriers within the social and built environment rather than within the individual. (1999, p. 245)

Standing, too, in advocating working in partnership with people with learning difficulties, also looks beyond the medical model and states:

> Working in partnership with people with learning difficulties demands for therapists far more than learning new techniques of treatment; it involves a willingness and capacity to respond imaginatively to every person as a unique individual and to help and support each person in the achievement of his or her own aspirations and desired lifestyle. (1999, p. 259)

TOWARDS EMANCIPATORY PRACTICE

Whatever your working knowledge of cultural diversity, it is essential that the 'voice' of clients, individual and collective, directs the provision of appropriate and culturally sensitive services. This applies through listening to individual clients whose daily experiences are likely to be fundamentally different to the experiences of therapists. It also applies through the consultation of organizations of people, such as people with learning difficulties, and people from black and ethnic minority communities, at every stage of service planning and implementation.

It has been increasingly recognized that the rationale of an inclusive strategy for disabled people who access health- and social-care services should be based on human rights. In terms of service practice, policy and procedure, disabled people's rights include: participating in care plans, audits and service provision; being consulted about practice health-care priorities; and having their needs considered. The campaign for civil rights legislation by disabled people and their supporters has a long history, both inside and outside parliament, and has been the major strategy of the disabled people's movement, in their struggle against institutionalized discrimination (Barnes 1991). Essentially this history dramatically illustrates the fundamental nature of institutionalized discrimination, and the concerted and collective efforts of a marginalized section of the population to break down discrimination. Campaigns in many countries (notably the USA, Canada and Australia) have led to civil-rights orientated legislation, and in the UK the political pressure culminated in the passing of the Disability Discrimination Act (DDA). Anti-discrimination and inclusion have increasingly underpinned changes in policy, provision and practice. Though the DDA has been criticized as limited in crucial ways (Swain et al. 2003), its implementation has a potentially important role to play in progress towards anti-discrimination. It states:

> Where a provider of services has a practice, policy or procedure which makes it impossible or unreasonably difficult for disabled people to make use of a service which he provides, or is prepared to provide, to other members of the public, it is his duty to take such steps as it is reasonable, in all circumstances of the case, for him to have to take in order to change that practice, policy or procedure so that it no longer has that effect. (DDA, Section 21)

Particular emphasis is placed on physical access to services and the provision of accessible information. There is a continuing need for trained interpreters, carefully matched to the client and his or her family, and independent of the particular organization. There is a need too for the provision of information about services in languages and forms accessible to all clients, potential clients and their families and assistants.

The employment of disabled, black and ethnic minority staff is of crucial importance. The discrimination faced by clients from minority groups can be faced too by members of staff and people from minority groups seeking employment, highlighting the importance of equal opportunity policies. There are many advantages to the employment of staff from minority groups. Black and ethnic minority staff, for instance, can communicate with clients in their own languages and can contribute to the evaluation of the adequacy of services, though it is important that such staff do not become restricted in their role to 'race experts' (Dominelli 2002).

A major strategy to changing disabling behaviours and practices is through the development of 'disability equality training' (DET). DET was originally devised by disabled people themselves and pioneered by a small group of disabled women in London (particularly by Jane Campbell, Micheline Mason and Kath Gillespie-Sells). In its strict sense DET originally referred to courses delivered only by tutors who have been trained by organizations of disabled people, in particular the Disability Resource Team in London and the Greater Manchester Coalition of Disabled People (Swain et al. 1998). These organizations train disabled people themselves to be trainers. DET courses are not about changing emotional responses to disabled people, but about challenging people's whole understanding of the meaning of 'disability'. They provide a basic introduction to the social model of disability and, in particular, the attitudinal, language, environmental and structural barriers that deny disabled people equal access to institutions and organizations. The following are the stated aims of courses run by disabled trainers who have themselves been trained through the work of the Disability Resource Team:

> A DET course will enable participants to identify and address discriminatory forms of practice towards disabled people. Through training they will find ways to challenge the organisational behaviour which reinforces negative myths and values and which prevents disabled people from gaining equality and achieving full participation in society. (Gillespie-Sells & Campbell 1991, p. 9)

Mason explains:

> It was designed to give service-providers the means to 'deconstruct' the medical model, understand the social model, and apply this new viewpoint to their particular area of influence or expertise . . . It is an attempt to help people realise how their perceptions of disability have become distorted, and to give them a brief insight into our own viewpoint on our situation. The goal is structural change. Through this training we have succeeded in creating a growing awareness amongst professionals that disability is a human rights issue. (2000, p. 109)

There are predominantly two types of disability training in practice: awareness and equality training. According to The Disability Rights Commission (www.drc-gb.org) the differences between the two are: awareness tends to 'focus on individual impairment' and 'will often involve simulation exercises'; equality, on the other hand, explores the concept of the social model of disability and would be carried out by a disabled person 'well versed in the social model'.

Swain & Lawrence (1994) suggest that DET is about: disability rather than impairment; improving attitudes by challenging the understanding of 'disability' and changing practices, rather than by attempting to change feelings towards disabled people; promoting a social rather than an individual model of disability; and the wider struggle for equal opportunities in both policies and practices. DET uses discussion-based methods for teaching and learning rather than simulation and is devised and delivered by disabled people.

Organizations may be becoming increasingly aware of their role in providing customer care for all their customers and clients. As Priestley (1999) points out, DET is now an established (albeit small) part of social work training courses in Britain. The Department of Health guidance on care management and assessment states that: 'The most effective way of demonstrating the centrality of users' needs and wishes will be by consulting users and carers over the training programme and inviting them to contribute to the training itself' (Department of Health et al. 1991, para. 106). Furthermore, the United Nations Standard Rules on the Equalization of Opportunities for People with Disabilities stipulates that disabled people's organizations should be involved in training development and that disabled people 'should be involved as teachers, instructors or advisers' (United Nations 1993, Rule 19.3). Awareness in Britain has been increased, in part, due to the DDA and also due to the awareness-raising initiatives being put in place by disabled individuals and disability groups.

Oliver & Barnes argue that the widespread use of DET as a radical new method of consciousness-raising has played a role in intensifying 'the pressure for nothing less than the full inclusion of disabled people with comprehensive civil rights legislation as the main vehicle for its achievement' (1998, p. 90).

There are dangers, however, in assuming that there has been progress. There is evidence to suggest that DET is not widely offered to professionals on an in-service basis (Swain et al. 1998). Furthermore, experience suggests that courses offered under the umbrella of DET differ quite widely in terms of their aims, who delivers them and how they are delivered. DET is not necessarily delivered by trainers who have been trained by organizations of disabled people. Also, some distance learning packages that claim to offer DET, for instance, are designed to raise awareness of impairment, even though this strategy has been rejected by organizations of disabled people and research evidence has repeatedly shown that such a strategy is ineffective in challenging social barriers.

There are similar arguments and issues about the provision of race equality training for therapists. French & Vernon, advocating race equality training, state:

> 'Race' equality training, when skilfully carried out by people from ethnic minority groups, can help people to become aware of their attitudes and behaviour in a relaxed and non-threatening environment. (1997, p. 66)

As in disability, there are different forms of training. Race awareness training resembles disability awareness training, while anti-racism awareness training corresponds to disability equality training. Anti-racism awareness training focuses on the social processes and racist power differentials existing between different ethnic minority groups, and links personal racism with structural racism; Dominelli states that: 'It also legitimates combining action aimed at eradicating racism with an appreciation of its effects' (1997, p.65).

One common element in all equality training is the use of language. In part this reflects the idea that language controls or constructs thinking. Sexism, ageism, homophobia, racism and disablism are framed within the very language we use. This has been characterized and degraded by some people as 'political correctness' (PC), often with reference to examples seen as trivial or fatuous (e.g. being criticized for offering black or white coffee). Use of language, however, is not simply about the legitimacy of words or phrases – what we are allowed to say or not say. As Thompson (1998) explains, language is a powerful vehicle within interactions between health- and social-care professionals and clients. He identifies a number of key issues:

- Jargon – the use of specialized language, creating barriers and mystification and reinforcing power differences
- Stereotypes – terms used to refer to people that reinforce presumptions, e.g. disabled people as 'sufferers'
- Stigma – terms that are derogatory and insulting, e.g. 'mentally handicapped'
- Exclusion – terms that exclude, overlook or marginalize certain groups, e.g. the term 'Christian name'
- Depersonalization – terms that are reductionist and dehumanizing, e.g. 'the elderly', 'the disabled' and even 'CPs' (to denote people with cerebral palsy).

Reflections

Perhaps less recognized is the use of disablist language. Make a list of words/phrases that you feel might be offensive to disabled people and alongside this list make another of more alternatives. If possible discuss this exercise with a disabled colleague and use your list to examine jargon, stereotyping, stigma, exclusion and depersonalization.

In this light, questions of the use of language go well beyond listing acceptable and unacceptable words, to examining ways of thinking that rationalize, legitimize and underline unequal therapist–client power relations.

To take just a few examples, sexist statements, for instance, stereotype women by attributing characteristics, occupations or exclusively subservient roles to women (for example, 'hysterical woman driver', 'devoted secretary'). The use of the word 'he' to refer to people in general has direct connotations of exclusion. The statement can usually be reworked using a person's name or job/role title (for example, the therapist, the client) or using the plural ('they', 'them', etc.). Other exclusive terms or phrases include 'mankind', 'best man for the job', 'chairman', 'spokesman', and 'manpower'. Likewise racism is expressed through racist language and stereotyping people from ethnic minorities. French & Sim state:

> Offensive terms, such as 'coloured' or 'half-caste', though once commonplace in everyday language, are no longer acceptable, and have been replaced by 'black' and 'mixed race'. Even the word 'immigrant' is frequently used in an abusive way. People from these groups are patronizingly overpraised for minor achievements, as if few others like them could achieve so much, and their ethnic origin is frequently referred to unnecessarily as in 'the brilliant black doctor'. (1993, p. 36)

The following are some suggestions from the British Council of Disabled People: use the term 'disabled person' rather than the word 'handicapped' or the word 'disabled' as a noun ('the disabled'). Do not refer to individuals by the medical conditions they have, for instance use 'a person with diabetes' rather than 'a diabetic'. Avoid some commonly used words: for 'victim' use 'person who has'/'person with'/'person who experienced'; 'crippled by', use 'person who has'/'person with'; 'suffering from', use 'person who has'/ 'person with'; 'afflicted by', use 'person who has'/'person with'; 'wheelchair bound', use 'wheelchair user'; 'mental handicap', use 'person with learning difficulties'; and 'invalid', use 'disabled person'.

This is not a definitive list. It includes, however, language that can not only be deeply offensive to disabled people, but also construct and maintain inequality. The use of the terms 'suffering' or 'afflicted', for instance, has clear connotations of helplessness, passivity, powerlessness and dependency on others.

Reflections

This exercise addresses initiating organizational change that, as Dominelli states:

> Is a complex task involving the orchestration of action seeking to remove individual racism, institutional racism and cultural racism in both policy and practice. (1997, pp. 145–146)

Our particular focus here is disablism, although the general principles are similar for racism, sexism and so on. The task is to formulate an action plan of constructive changes in policy and practice in your organization that will contribute to the gathering momentum for change in the social, economic, and political position of disabled people. The plan should have five steps:

1. SUBJECT – What is the broad area that you have picked out for improvement?
2. GOALS – What specific targets do you wish to achieve?
3. PROBLEMS – What barriers are you going to encounter?
4. SOLUTIONS – How do you plan to deal with the barriers?
5. ACTIVITIES – List in sequence the steps to bring about the desired change and indicate the time period.

In formulating this action plan it is essential that: disabled people are involved at every stage (clients, disabled colleagues, and representatives of local organizations of disabled people); the plan reflects a social rather than an individual model of disability; the formulation of the action plan is a collaborative activity, within which participants develop ways of working together and supporting each other; and participants develop their knowledge and understanding of disability to enable them to recognize and challenge the discriminatory language and the visual images, discriminatory policies and practices that help to perpetuate the inequality of disabled people.

PART 4

In professional education

Part 4 looks at the implications for education and training itself. The two chapters are written by Jim Clark, who is himself an educator. In Chapter 11 he considers what is involved in working with professional groups, including therapists, to develop their understanding and practice in terms of enabling relationships. He develops the ideas in the chapter around extracts from a story of two tutors, himself and a colleague, and a group of students who are involved in a course on enabling relationships in professional contexts. Extracts from this story are presented to allow you to consider the issues of working with groups, including: issues of sharing practice; ethics and principles; and after session discussions. Jim suggests that education is about reflective practice. This reflective practice needs to be considered carefully for all professions as a basis of education rather than training. In the following chapter, Jim explores the ingredients that can underpin the detailed planning of a programme. He builds upon the story told in the previous chapter to examine, for instance: ethically based principles, procedures and outcomes; time – looking back to look forward; design of activities; and management of programmes in creating enabling learning environments. He suggests that the tutor in this setting needs to be a committed reflective practitioner with a strong understanding of the principle at the heart of reflective practice in trying to develop an understanding of processes of enabling relationships that can be used by professionals. The outcome should enable them to be better practitioners within their own fields of professional responsibility.

Chapter 11

Enabling relationships in professional education

Jim Clark

> What one knows, in a final sense, one knows about oneself. Who one is, is inextricably bound up with who one is known to be. (Salmon 1980, p. 5)

In this chapter I will be considering what is involved in working with professional groups, including therapists, to develop their understanding and practice in terms of enabling relationships. As with other sections of this book it is intended to be interactive and create a dialogue between the text and the readers. The readers have the power to make sense of the text and the ideas contained within. I recognize that readers use books in all sorts of ways and may not have started with the introduction and followed each chapter through to this point. In acknowledging this, the chapter incorporates ideas expressed earlier and will also refer the reader to other chapters for more detailed discussion of ideas. If you can create the opportunity to share your thoughts and ideas with another person as you engage in the reflective activities provided, these will give opportunities to examine your own views and those of others. In the process of engaging in the reflective activities you could be building a course booklet.

I develop the ideas in the chapter around extracts from a story of two tutors, myself and a colleague, and a group of students who are involved in a course on enabling relationships in professional contexts. The extracts from this story are there to allow you and I to consider the issues of working with groups, so that we have some images of people and practice in our minds around which we can think about the issues, theories and practice.

SHARING PRACTICE

Working with any group in a professional educational context can be exciting, challenging, frightening, and worrying. These feelings that I often have, as workshop leader and educator, are still the same after all these years of working. There is always a feeling of tentativeness in beginning this work with a new group. I am sure that all professional educators experience some of these feelings, as well as the stories that we collect about good and not so good sessions. Along with these, we remember the members of those sessions who worked well or not so well, were indifferent or became excited about the ideas, but these all feed both our reflection and our practice. It is with that feeling of tentativeness that I begin to share my thinking and very public reflection on practice that writing a chapter like this demands. So who am I?

Professionally I started my career as a primary and early-years teacher. I then moved on to work within a local education authority as a part of the advisory service before becoming a university tutor. I am currently involved in researching and teaching in the field of arts, creativity and early-years education. I have taught and teach on courses, which have as their content thinking and learning, the arts, creativity and enabling relationships. I have a commitment and interest in the ways in which an anti-discriminatory way of working and living can be developed. The self and identity are central to this and I believe core to enabling relationships.

I do not want to create 'the model' for practice and I recognize the tensions in setting out a model for practice, in that it could become prescriptive. Therefore, I will use the word 'approach', which better suits the fluidity and flexibility of the way many other professional educators and I work. The ideas explored are aimed at helping professionals to reflect on their current practice or to develop new ways of working, through considering this approach and engaging in the reflections. I would hope that resonance between my reflections about what the tutors try to do, the voices of our students and the individual reader's reflections on this work can aid the development of future practice, either as a tutor or as one of our students.

The ways of working derive from the set of core principles that have grown out of the developing theory and the constantly evolving practice reflected in the earlier chapters. I focus on these principles and the approach in Chapter 12. Here my concern is to present the opportunity to reflect on evidence and experiences, and discuss the key emerging issues from these personal experiences. The ideas represent a moment marked in my continuing personal and professional development in supporting individuals and groups to understand the complexities of enabling positive relationships with others. My thinking has moved on to focus on the centrality of the processes of communication in developing enabling relationships in professional settings. The ideas are based upon the very real social interactions that occur between individuals and have often derived from our intuitive practice (Atkinson & Claxton 2000) into explicitly expressed practice. They include those moments when an idea of what should happen next just appears as I am working in a session. Then after the session, when reflecting on what occurred, I think 'that bit where we . . . that went well – I'll have to remember to include that next time!', but I know that next time it won't be the same. What was described in the introduction as 'stumbling' provides our starting point.

A STARTING POINT

The other day a colleague, who was asking me about this book and what enabling relationships were all about, suddenly stated, 'the theory is all very well and I can *sign up* to it but putting it into practice in some classrooms, with some students, can be another thing altogether!'. Having just finished a particularly difficult meeting, I felt I knew what my colleague meant. In the difficult meeting my ability to listen, *really listen* with complete unconditional regard to the other's perspective was, to say the least, challenged. When reflecting upon what had occurred in the meeting I realized, once again, that the complexity occurring in that social interaction was the construction of meaning within the dialogue. I was not putting the theoretical ideas I had explored in the past into practice, but was once again engaged in a much more dynamic encounter where the theory, the ideas and the meaning were being created in the moment by two relational beings.

A STORY

The story I tell is developed from working with groups over a period of time. It includes reflections on that work through both discussion between a colleague and myself, and our notes and memories. Through meeting some real people, voices and events, you and I can reflect on the key issues, work and ideas about enabling relationships in professional contexts.

Extracts from working with the group

I begin with an account of a group that have come together to work with my colleague and I on an enabling relationship course. The course, based on the ideas in this book, took place over 10 weeks in 3-hour sessions within a continuing professional development programme. It always draws from a multi-professional base and is strengthened by that mix.

Who are they?

This particular group included two further education tutors; a university librarian; a teacher; a nurse tutor from the university; six therapists, including speech and language and physio; eight nurses with a variety of professional experience; and a university lecturer who happens to be a colleague. The group as a whole has a wide range of experiences and a wide range of reasons for coming on the course.

> Tutor: So lets make a start.
> Group member: I like to know what's going to happen in sessions when I'm on a course. I don't like surprises, I don't think it's fair. It's the same in our centre. We like to tell the clients what's happening and what's happening next. It makes them happier.

Why are we here?

At the start of session one we always ask the group why they are here and what they hope to get from the time we will be working together. This not only enables an insight to be gained into their intentions, but also will allow us to refine our planning to better meet their particular needs. One said that she was here because the course sounded interesting and she wondered what enabling relationships might be about. Another had not seen any other course being offered at that time that he fancied in order to get more points towards his master of education degree. The therapists were here as a part of their updating programme run by the local health authority.

This subgroup had a mix of views about the value of being on the course including two who stated that they could not see the point of developing relationships with patients beyond finding out what was wrong. Another shared the view that she 'didn't think it was their job to get involved in counselling'. The quiet member of this group thought it would be useful in getting to work with the patients in a closer and more focused way:

> I want to be able to share my thinking about working with my clients and my colleagues and see if I can make it easier for all of us.

The teacher had discussed the course with me when I had been into the school to do a session on working with a variety of professionals in educational settings. He was interested in some of the activities and discussions that had occurred. One of the further education tutors felt it might help him support his students and get on better with some of his 'difficult staff'. The other tutor had read John Swain's book on counselling skills and thought that it might be interesting to come and work with us.

Baggage

In further discussion it was clear that the group had a wide range of experiences and were bringing all sorts of 'baggage' with them:

> Wouldn't it be interesting to know why we all say what we say and respond like we do?

> At work it's as if there's a culture of behaving in certain ways to our clients, I can't remember being told or learning it, it just happened.

> When you talked about the 'baggage' that we carry around being like a bag full of 'stuff' that makes us who we are and act and relate as we do, it didn't make sense at first but now I've read the handout and reflected I think it's useful.

Some of the 'baggage' that they are clearly carrying is associated with what this course is about and what they expect from it. They ranged in their needs and desires. Some wanted skills they could use, 'I want some training in using techniques to get on better with my patients'. Another said, 'I want to understand how people relate to each other and how to improve and support them in their workplace'. Thus indicating an often-occurring dilemma between training and education, which I discuss later in this chapter.

Ethics and principles

> If I had known when I was starting to work with you two and the group that I would have to explore and face so many things about myself and

how I related to others and how they saw me I might never have started! But I don't regret it, well not now.

In part of the session we always made clear the set of ethical principles that we see as underpinning our practice in working with groups. These are developed from principles that should underpin good practice in professional settings. The teacher commented that:

> We had a meeting the other day to reflect on what our key principles might be, that caused a lot of discussion and I thought oops! We haven't got a real one. We've just relied on the curriculum documentation.

This enabled us to discuss issues relating to ethical principles underpinning our practice. Another group member added:

> Trying to think about the principles that were underpinning our practice at work and decide how they were made real in our behaviours to each other and our students was difficult.

My colleague and I always made the ethical issues, code and rules for the series of sessions very explicit. We made it clear to the group that for us the ethical code and key rules are concerned with enabling the participants to develop a level of trust that will support them to feel that they can talk, discuss and reflect in an open way:

> When you work with us I've never seen you put anyone down, which feels good. It has helped me to be able to test out ideas in front and with others and not feel stupid.

It is only by having a context in which this can occur that any of us can develop our reflective practice and the understanding and skills that are needed to be able to sustain this in practice.

The next phase in the work is to move on to consider the concept of enabling relationships in professional settings. During this session the group was introduced to ideas about understanding self and the way that, as individuals, we communicate and interact with others in our professional settings. This leads us to discussions of the concept of 'us' and 'we'. Here are some of the points expressed by the group:

> I sense I know what you mean. It's there but I don't have to think about it to know. Wouldn't it be interesting to know why we all say what we say and respond like we do?

We were intending to get the group members to begin to look at the ideas of what we take for granted about ourselves and our ways of interacting with others and how others might interpret us. Having talked a little about self and about taking account of our own feelings, understandings, beliefs and principles, we moved on to look at how our awareness of self also develops from being aware of ourselves from within relationships. Key to this is being able to monitor the responses that others make to what we offer, say or do:

What has been really useful, I know we have only had ten weeks, working together, is the way, although we've done a lot, look at the size of my portfolio, but there has always seemed to be time, we haven't rushed things.

After session discussions

Our discussions after the individual sessions are and have been very important to my colleague and me. They provide mutual support and critical friendship, which both challenges us and sustains us. We often reassure one another about what each of us has done in the session. It is good to share the positive as well:

I thought it was interesting this evening when you were getting them to think again about the incidents from their own practice and trying to get them to envisage another perspective on the incident.

When we all get talking, I feel that I'm really involved and concerned with what we are exploring.

When we all got talking this evening I wondered if (Alan) was resisting some of the ideas and I thought that he was becoming isolated and I wasn't sure how to draw him back in . . .

He didn't want to move from his management role and see the experience from another perspective . . . I thought it was best to leave it in the end.

There are some times when we are working that there is a real dialogue going between us all as a group, even you two. It feels as if there is a real commitment. It feels supportive.

These discussions are also very important in enabling us to:

- draw on mutual support and criticism in a supportive and enabling environment
- consider the specific needs of the group and the individuals in the group; these are always very different
- reflect upon the process of the session
- plan the next session by analyzing the previous session against the principles that we hold at the heart of our work on enabling relationships.

Sometimes and if possible we would hold these straight after sessions and, if not, at a time before the next session. We both use journals to keep notes of things that might have been said by participants, our own thoughts on sessions and ideas for future work with the group. In these reflections we would look at what happened in relation to:

- our ethical principles
- our overall intentions
- the processes of working

- how we had related to the group and how the individuals had related in the group both to us and each other
- the content we use in supporting the process of learning
- how we have worked in creating enabling relationships.

Extract from journal

> There was a discussion arising from the exercise about how we perceive ourselves and how others perceive us . . . wasn't comfortable about this exercise and didn't want to talk. I was pleased that Jim spoke to me after the session. What was said was important.
>
> When we did the exercise I wasn't comfortable at first with talking about it. I prefer to work things out on my own. I think it's because I didn't know you at first. I think there was a tension that I felt that some of the group were beginning to see this personal reflection as individualistic and had to ensure that the group had a sense of this as being embedded in relationships and context.
>
> You two are always very quiet in sessions with us aren't you? I don't mean you stay quiet, but you act in a quiet way, you listen and often somehow it feels as if all the ideas and thinking is ours.

One of the ongoing discussions that we have is about creating an enabling environment: one in which the group can work and feel safe enough to explore aspects of enabling relationships to ensure that learning occurs for the group and the tutor. This has many aspects to it including the emotional, cognitive and physical. We have to ensure that the group becomes committed to the work that they are doing and are enabled to reflect and move forward. The approach has to have 'a sense of soul'.

Having introduced the story I will now share my thinking about enabling relationships in professional educational contexts by using examples from the story to discuss the issues that are raised by these components. The first issue is whether we are involved in training or educating.

TRAINING OR EDUCATION?

> I want some training in using techniques to get on better with my patients.

I have, therefore, suggested that education be about reflective practice. This reflective practice needs to be considered carefully for all professions as a basis of education rather than training. We will, therefore, be considering reflective practice throughout this chapter. Engaging in the process of reflective practice is complex and if we are to develop this reflective practice in others we have to be using reflection in our own practice. How such reflective approaches can be established within a learning programme has often been a tricky area. Ross & Hannay remind us that unfortunately:

Too frequently the rationale for reflective teaching is expounded through expository techniques and a technical enquiry approach. (1986, p. 9)

This is a key point for us in thinking about how to work with groups to develop their reflective practice. They go on to state that:

> ...the university classroom must become not only the venue for transmitting traditional knowledge on teacher education but also a laboratory where such practices are modelled, experienced, and reflected upon. Such a truly reflective model needs to be firmly grounded in critical theory by incorporating the application of principles, not procedures, in the investigation ... (1986, p. 9)

Ghaye & Lillyman (2000) usefully discussed the impact of ideas to do with reflective practice as a way of being. They suggest that this growth in reflective approaches to practice is a:

> ...reaction against the view of professionals as 'technicians' who merely carry out what others, removed from practice, want them to do. (2000, p. 35)

Our focus on human interaction, reflective and emancipatory practice acknowledges that individuals in these professions are more than technicians and are engaged in education.

Dewey (1933) highlighted the idea of 'artful skills'. I would see the professionals as being in the business of using reflection as a way of helping them to use their artful skills with others in meaningful ways that enable positive outcomes. Understanding the art in what the individual professional does is, I feel, key to seeing the process as more than training. Training suggests the possibility of using a manual, a text or demonstration. However, the art is developed through dialogue with others into an understanding of the complexities of the role, the self and others. As Ghaye & Lillyman point out when trying to define reflective practice: 'Reflection can therefore be about many things' (2000, p. 35).

Reflections

Having read the discussion above consider how you see your own role when working with your students or trainees. Do you see yourself as being in the business of education or training? How do other colleagues see themselves in relation to the education or training debate? If you are a student you might reflect on whether certain of your tutors fit the training or education divide. Discuss with a colleague how you both see yourselves and why. Another interesting aspect to this is whether our students see themselves as engaging in a process of training or an educational process. Using the above material construct a paragraph or two on this issue that might be in the introduction to a course booklet on enabling relationships.

Therefore, in considering the organization of workshops about enabling relationships, it has to be about reflections on the self, others and 'us' as was highlighted in Chapter 1.

As part of the process of examining and constructing our working practice, and the theoretical underpinning to that approach, it is important to explore the relational self.

RELATIONAL SELVES – TAKEN FOR GRANTED REALITIES

> I sense I know what you mean. It's there but I don't have to think about it to know.

> Wouldn't it be interesting to know why we all say what we say and respond like we do?

> I don't know why I said that.

It is time to think about the people that we work with and what they bring with them; their taken for granted ideas and their 'baggage'. The challenge is to find a way of working that allows both ourselves as professional educators and our students to examine some of the aspects of our tacit or taken for granted *ideas* about ourselves as individuals in constant interaction with others. From this examination we can try to help each other to develop those qualities highlighted by Ghaye & Lillyman (2000) above. This tacit knowledge underpins the ways in which we interact with others and our responses to situations we find ourselves in. We have all heard someone say, 'I don't know why I said that' or 'I don't know why I did that', and sometimes have said it ourselves. Such responses are often a result of tacit knowledge or understandings we have. We have to enable individuals to read the way that they interact with others. They have to be supported in understanding the messages that we all give out and those that are given in response.

It would be useful to pause a moment in our discussion and briefly outline tacit knowledge. The term tacit knowledge was used in 1976, for the first time, by Michael Polanyi to describe the way that we become so skilled in carrying out certain actions in our personal and professional lives, that we no longer have to think about them and just know them. Claxton (2000) describes these varieties of intuitive operations and ways of thinking as 'ways of knowing'. They are often habitual, like being able to ride a bike or responding to certain individuals in certain ways, for example the ritual of greeting that we use towards a partner when arriving home at the end of the day.

In the case of emancipatory or anti-discriminatory practice, as discussed in Chapter 10, our communication affects the way we behave, within our professional context, to our clients or students. In developing enabling relationships we have to be able to examine these taken-for-granted understandings or realities and reflect, re-present and see them as new. This 'seeing as new' enables us to challenge our interactions with, and behaviours towards, one another. The basis for this has to be through reflective practice as described in Chapter 6. As Thompson reminds us very clearly:

... the world we live in is an extremely complex one that presents major challenges for any individuals or groups that seek to change the status quo. What we must recognise, then, is the need to find a constructive balance between the extremes of cynicism and defeatism on the one hand, and a naïve idealism on the other. Finding and maintaining that balance can be a difficult and demanding task. (1998, p. 5)

Building our understanding of, and becoming involved in enabling relationships is both difficult and demanding. This is particularly true in talking about promoting equality. As Thompson (1998) recognizes, change in a professional context is extremely complicated. The challenge is to find ways of making this tacit activity explicit. Through this process we can make explicit the purpose and shape of our practice, and allow others and ourselves to examine it and reflect upon it. It is risky for the individual and can become both uncomfortable and deskilling before it becomes empowering for others and ourselves. Nias stated that teachers on enquiry-based courses, if not properly supported by the course tutors, can be left '... deskilled, disoriented, isolated and rendered impotent by their experience' (1988, p. 10).

BAGGAGED SELVES

At work it's as if there's a culture of behaving in certain ways to our clients. I can't remember being told or learning it. It just happened.

When you talked about the 'baggage' that we carry around being like a bag full of 'stuff' that makes us who we are and act and relate as we do, it didn't make sense at first but now I've read the handout and reflected I think it's useful.

Working in any setting can be challenging because of the 'cultural baggage' that we all bring with us. This also extends to the baggage that the setting or training institution has. Baggage here means the ideological, political, moral, social, cultural beliefs and understandings that we carry around with us and that are made real through the way we present ourselves, interact and the language we use. As Friere states:

Human existence cannot be silent, nor can it be nourished by false words, but only true words, with which men (sic) transform the world. To exist, humanly, is to name the world, to change it. Once named, the world reappears to the namers as a problem and requires of them a new naming. (1972, pp. 60, 61).

The words we use and the language and meaning they create are part of our socially interactive experience informed by and contributing to this baggage or cultural rucksack.

This, therefore, has to be our starting point as it is the only place we can begin. To work towards enabling relationships will mean working with this baggage and often confronting aspects of our practices, both personal and professional. This will, in the process, become an exploration of the often hidden internal contradictions that exist in all of us. A process of unravelling these hidden contradictions that exist in our discourse or practice, as Nightingale & Cromby suggest, could allow us to 'destabilise, subvert and resist dominant forms of knowledge' (1999, p. 226). In developing an approach to working in enabling relationships we all have to be willing to open up our cultural rucksacks and examine the contents. As Berger points out:

> Only an understanding of internalisation makes sense of the incredible fact that most external controls work most of the time for most people in a society. Society not only controls our movements, but also shapes our identity, our thoughts and our emotions. The structures of society become the structure of our own consciousness. Society does not stop at the surface of our skins. Society penetrates us as much as it envelops us. (1966, p. 140)

We need to recognize the way that the stories that exist in many forms and 'penetrate our skins' not only control us but also allow us to create our identity and account for our actions in our world. We need, as educators and professional therapists, to know that the cultural structures of what it means to be a therapist can be very strong and also get under our skin. They form the models of what a therapist is, how the relationships between therapist and client should be framed, how we should relate to other professionals and, more importantly within this discussion, how we as tutors have created the approaches that we use for learning and reflection.

Sometimes it is difficult to recall our taken-for-granted behaviours, but it becomes important to be able to reflect upon these if we are going to be able to see how we can build enabling relationships. With the ideas above in mind, and still concentrating on the people involved, let us move on to look at learning and its influence on the tutors and the students.

Reflections

The idea of cultural stories of how we should behave, getting under our skin, and becoming a part of our 'taken-for-granted reality' is interesting and worth reflecting upon. Take a moment to think through a greetings ritual you use with a partner or family member. Now think of the greetings ritual you use towards a colleague. What are the elements that make up these two rituals? What are the emotional and interpersonal attitudes that are displayed in this 'greetings ritual'? Reflect upon these two rituals and consider how others might read those behaviours and words.

LEARNING SELVES

The way the sessions go on this course are nothing like I thought they would be. I thought you would tell us more.

The development and learning that occur within any session is based upon a contract between the tutor and the individual students within the group. This may not always be expressed as an explicit contract, but rather remains as an implicit agreement in which both parties play their role. This contract allows for potential learning to occur. I would contend that learning and, indeed, teaching cannot be divorced from, or considered independently of the personal relationships that occur within a group, or between individuals and the tutor. Without this aspect being present in the working relationships, the individuals may not be willing to take the risks required to reflect and transform current understandings into new learning. Learners will have differing views of what learning is for and/or its value. In a study into learning in higher education Martin & Ramsden (1987, p. 155) use Slajo's (1979) conceptions to learning. Slajo usefully accompanies these conceptions with voices of the students.

Conception 1: learning as the increase of knowledge

The main feature of this first category is its vagueness, in the sense that what is given in the answers is merely a set of synonyms for the word learning.

Conception 2: learning as memorizing

The meaning of learning is to transfer units of information or pieces of knowledge, or facts from a teacher or book, into the head.

Conception 3: learning as the acquisition of facts or procedures that can be retained and/or utilized in practice

Some facts and principles are considered to be practically useful and, as a consequence, they are given special attention and remembered for a long time:

> Yes to learn so that you know it and so that you can make use of it. It shouldn't be just learning something, which disappears immediately after you've learnt it, but you should be able to make use of it even after a while.

Conception 4: learning as the abstraction of meaning

With this conception the nature of what is learned is changed. Learning is no longer an activity of reproduction, but a process of abstracting meaning:

> For me learning does not mean that you should learn all those petty details but instead it means learning about a course of events and how things have developed and reasoning within my subject but it does not mean sitting down and memorizing trifles such as dates and such things.

Reflections

Looking at the list of conceptions decide which you as a learner and a tutor find as the most powerful in relation to learning? Which most closely underpins the practice arising in this book?

Conception 5: learning as an interpretative process aimed at the understanding of reality

This conception is similar to conception 4, but there is an additional suggestion that learning should help you interpret the reality in which you live. What is interesting is if you ask the student groups you work with about their own conceptions of learning you will find they make responses under these categories.

In working with individuals and groups in the area of enabling relationships, with its focus upon reflective and emancipatory practice, I really want my students to perceive the learning that 'should help you interpret the reality in which you live'. With this in mind we move onto enabling environments as a context for learning.

ENABLING ENVIRONMENTS FOR LEARNING

There are some times when we are working that there is a real dialogue going between us all as a group, even you two. It feels as if there is a real commitment, it feels supportive.

When we all get talking, I feel that I'm really involved and concerned with what we are exploring.

If we are going to work with a group of individuals to develop an understanding of enabling relationships then we, as tutors, have to create an enabling environment with the opportunity for the processes of enabling, or enhancing, relationships between the participants: professionals and clients. This environment would be where individuals can come together, share, discuss and reflect on their own and others' feelings, views and understandings. It would be an environment where reflection with a sense of soul can occur for the students. An environment that provides an atmosphere in which the students will feel comfortable to take risks and where they have a sense of ownership over what is happening. As Jennings & Kennedy (1996, p. 83) in citing Kolb (1984) indicated, there are three key points in thinking about learning:

1. We learn best when personally involved in the learning experience.
2. Knowledge of any kind has more significance when we learn it through our own initiative, insight or discovery.
3. Learning is best when we are committed to aims that we have been involved in setting, when our participation with others is valued and when there is a supportive framework in which to learn.

Chapter **12**

Enabling relationships: the ingredients for practice

Jim Clark

INTRODUCTION

This chapter explores the *ingredients* that can underpin the detailed planning of a programme. I am building upon the story told in the previous chapter. Although I will be discussing the ingredients, the chapter does not produce the recipe! You will produce your own as you take the ingredients and blend them into your work. As Ashcroft & Foreman-Peck state, we need to build '. . . from experience and evidence, rather than to learn certain "recipes" for action' (1994, p. 3). As the reader you can reflect upon your own experiences as you engage with the ideas or use the experience and evidence presented in the previous chapter. The focus here then is to explore the key ingredients that can be used to create an enabling environment for the learners. The chapter may also help you to develop the handbook started in Chapter 11.

THE KEY INGREDIENTS

Within the approach used for this work there are certain key ingredients that the tutor needs to be constantly drawing upon to enable the opportunity for the group they are working with to move to an understanding of how to create, develop, sustain and reflect upon enabling relationships. The approach brings together the following ingredients:

- ethically based principles, procedures and outcomes
- the process of working – an approach to practice
- interacting with the group
- management and facilitation of sessions
- time – looking back to look forward
- what kind of tutor(s) is needed
- the programme: towards felt understanding.

The rest of this chapter discusses each ingredient drawing on ideas presented in the earlier chapters in the book.

ETHICALLY BASED PRINCIPLES, PROCEDURES AND OUTCOMES

> The theory is all very well and I can signup to it but putting it into practice in some classrooms, with some students, can be another thing altogether!

> We had a meeting the other day to reflect on what our key principles might be, that caused a lot of discussion and I thought oops! We haven't got a real one. We've just relied on the curriculum documentation.

Developing ethically based principles, procedures and outcomes in the field of enabling relationships is not easy. It's even harder to stick to them. Unlike training models and fixed recipes, we are dealing with, and examining directly, the living interactions of individuals within socially complex situations. In helping these individuals to develop enabling relationships, they have to be willing to examine aspects of their own feelings, beliefs and behaviours, and share some of these with each other. They will be asked to problematize their own practice. These following principles are adapted from Ghaye & Ghaye (1998, p. 66). Problematizing practice can involve an element of discomfort, even threat, as we look at ourselves and our working environment. It is far easier to accept our current circumstances and adopt the line of least resistance. This could be seen in the therapists' encounters with Ken Walker, in the case study from Chapter 9, where the medical model was used to hide behind rather than listen.

As a result of problematizing practice, there is a need to reflect on what you, or others, perceive to be inadequacies of your professional practice, your strengths and how to nourish and sustain existing good practice. What were the inadequacies in the therapists' actions in Ken Walker's case?

It is not mandatory to introduce new and different perspectives from the outside. However, it is important, through collective action, to reflect upon the values on which practice is taking place and to examine the real possibilities which practice, on this occasion, chooses to ignore or cannot enact. What values underpinned the practice in the Walker case study?

Problematizing therapy or any other practice, including being a tutor teaching enabling relationships, means we reflect upon what is happening and why, what our professional or educational intentions are and why we hold them.

Students will have their beliefs and ways of being challenged and asked to see the world from a variety of differing perspectives, as was presented in the case study in Chapter 9. As discussed earlier, this can be risky and sometimes breach our comfort zones. The comfort zone is the mental and or physical space within which we operate and feel comfortable and not threatened. Let us begin by looking at ethical principles and procedures.

Ethical principles and procedures

In this section I set out and discuss the ethical principles that I try to adhere to in working with others: the first of our ingredients. In building these principles, I acknowledge the two critical approaches outlined earlier in Chapter 6.

1. An approach that takes as the starting point the challenging of discrimination and oppression by empowering individuals to take greater control of their lives.
2. Critical practice based upon open-mindedness, which takes account of different perspectives, experiences and assumptions.

These critical approaches underpin my practice and, therefore, have to inform the ethical principle, action principles, and procedures and outcome principles. In exploring principles here, I hold to Dewey's notion of open-mindedness that:

> . . . recognise[s] the possibility of error even in the beliefs that are dearest to us. (1933, p. 29)

I also accept that, as Rowland reminds us:

> Educational theories and models, like analogies, should be treated with caution. (1993, p. 16)

These principles will, therefore, inform our: enabling relationships, critical reflection, and empowerment and emancipation.

These principles and procedures have to underpin my work from the first meeting of a group, establishing the working relationships, the rules of working together, the way I manage, the way we organize as a group, the way we plan the tasks for and within the group, and how we reflect upon the experience. The recipe takes shape when all of these ingredients are in place. We only know if the recipe works after we have made it! This leads me to my central ethical principle: to ensure that all those with whom I work are enabled to have a voice and to be able to share their thoughts, feelings and understandings about self and others through a mutually respectful dialogue. The dialogue is supported by unconditional positive regard that enables everyone to feel safe and valued as a person. Growing out from this central principle is a series of other principles for actions, behaviours, and outcomes both within and arising out of the session activities.

Principles for our actions and behaviours

The following principles inform actions and behaviours, particularly with groups in sessions. Through these actions and behaviours with my students I attempt to:

- facilitate the recognition and questioning of power relations, structures and ideologies that limit people's freedom
- promote mutual understanding and awareness of others' preferences, wishes and needs through open two-way communication
- promote people's prediction and control over decision-making processes that shape their lives
- facilitate reflection through critical examination of the practice/process of human relationships in contexts to examine assumptions, values and biases

- develop an understanding of reflective and emancipatory practice and a critical stance towards debates about theory and practice
- facilitate, through actively working in partnership with groups, a collaborative approach to organization, planning, delivery and evaluation of work in sessions and our workplace activities.

Principles for outcomes

With the above ethical principles, the following underpin the outcomes for students. Students will be able, through personal reflection individually and through dialogue, to promote an understanding of self and others, and of the values both embedded in society's structure and constructed in interpersonal communication and relationships. They will also be able to promote people's understanding of struggles against repression and 'man-made' sufferings, and support the removal of barriers to equal opportunities and full participatory citizenship for all.

These principles and procedures for working create both the aims for my work and also the outcomes of the experiences. Through my work with students I explore as the content of the work: the assumptions underlying perspectives relating to concepts of 'self', communication, and relationships and their implications for working within educational and professional contexts; the assumptions underlying the concepts of 'empowerment' and 'partnership' in educational and professional settings; the examination of the organization and management of interpersonal communication and enabling relationships within educational and professional settings; at the personal/interpersonal level, the processes of communication in forming and maintaining relationships in the educational and professional settings.

Reflections

In thinking about your own practice as an educator, which of the above ethical principles would you adhere to, which ones would you want to modify? On a sheet of paper write out the ones you think are of value and exist in your practice. Rewrite any that you feel you want to change.

Write out any additional principles you feel are not expressed in the list above but do or would exist if you were in a training role. Consider the ethical nature of your principles and procedures. You might like to use the following as a guide to discussion.

What is in an ethical code? Think about ethical behaviours, agreed explicit rules, what this work is and what it isn't, and how we will work together.

Now write these as a section of the evolving handbook. In developing this and reflecting on this section you may want to visit or revisit the chapter on ethics for support or to develop your understanding.

As a result of this engagement, I hope to have empowered the students to be able to analyze the power relationships and structures in communication and in the relationships that shape the decision-making processes, in particular, in the educational and professional contexts. From this I engage them in the processes of planning and evaluating strategies for improving the organization and management of relationships and communication within their own professional settings. Out of this I support them in developing their communication skills in working in partnership with and empowering clients and colleagues.

Having explored the central ethical principles, procedures and outcomes that underpin my approach I will share how these work in practice with groups and individuals.

THE PROCESS OF WORKING – AN APPROACH TO PRACTICE

If I had known when I was starting to work with you two and the group that I would have to explore and face so many things about myself and how I related to others and how they saw me I might never have started. But I don't regret it, well not now.

When I came to the first session and you talked about ethical principles and that discussions about settings being kept in the room I thought, 'oh God I'm on one of those therapy or counselling events.' Sorry no offence meant to the therapists here.

I want to be able to share my thinking about working with my clients and my colleagues and see if I can make it easier for all of us.

In this section on an approach to practice I set out the key areas for consideration. It is worth reminding ourselves at this point that what we are interested in here is the development of enabling relationships and not with acting as a counsellor. As Swain points out, 'perhaps even more questionable is the possibility of "dabbling in counselling", that is delving into client space personal lives without their consent and against their wishes' (1995, p. 34). What I am acknowledging here is that aspects of counselling can be used and adapted to enable us to operate within our professional lives with others. I am using counselling skills not in the sense that counsellors might use them within formal counselling sessions, but on a more 'ad hoc' basis as a part of our practice as professionals. In drawing upon these skills and understandings we are operating from a humanistic set of principles that enable us to consider each individual's uniqueness. The focus is not on developing counselling skills, but upon the relational aspects of being professionals with our respective client groups. As Gergen writes:

. . . the conception of relational being reduces the debilitating gap between self and other, the sense of oneself as alone and the other as alien and untrustworthy. Whatever we are, from the present standpoint, is either directly or indirectly with others. . . . We are made up of each other. . . . we are mutually constituting. (1999, pp. 137–138)

Our focus in supporting and developing practice has to be on these relationships that exist between people, rather than the skills that one person might use on another. Salmon (1980) argues that what we know about our world is what one ultimately knows about oneself. Therefore, we cannot disentangle ourselves from the lives of others as we operate as relational beings. As I said earlier our work in enabling relationships is as much about us as it is our students. The process of working with people and the approach to practice has at its heart the ways that the students and I interact with one another.

Interacting with the group

When you gave us things to do or think about you left us to work at it and only interfered when we asked or you perceived that there was a need to.

When you work with us I've never seen you put anyone down, which feels good. It has helped me to be able to test out ideas in front and with others and not feel stupid.

The ways of working are based on principles of empowerment, anti-discriminatory and reflective practice. This has to be reflected in the ways in which we interact and work with the group. I recognize that my own practice has developed in context, as I have worked alongside others in workshops, seminars, tutorials and meetings. Ideas have evolved through our social interactions in sessions with trainees, therapists and tutors, trying to construct what Gergen calls 'collaborative classrooms' (1999, p. 182). For me the classroom should be a live, socially interactive environment in which issues relating to human relations, and the ideas and practice relating to enabling relationships, can be openly and supportively explored. Importantly for us, Gergen states:

. . . reliance on monologue not only fails to take advantage of the multiple skills that students bring to the class, but there is little opportunity for the students to appropriate subject matter in their own terms. There is little opportunity for them to take what is useful from the material in ways that can enrich their particular circumstances; more colloquially, they fail 'to own the material'. (1999, p. 182)

If the approach that I am proposing is to be of use to the students, then the classroom must be a place of dialogue leading to empowerment and ownership of ideas that can become part of their ongoing practice. The work of Schön (1987) on reflective practice is important here. Schön showed in his various writings that a range of professionals operated by using their current understandings, beliefs, values and attitudes to look at a situation, engage in a solution finding process, reflect upon this solution and re-evaluate their practice. In so doing they change their current understandings, beliefs, values and attitudes.

I am, therefore, moving on to explore the key components of the process of working with groups on enabling relationships. The area of interest here is in the way tutor(s) can enable groups to become reflective and use their experience, knowledge and understandings of self and others to critically reflect upon situations. As a result of this process of reflection they can transform their understanding of themselves and others, and are able to recognize the ways in which they can create enabling relationships within a variety of professional contexts. Ghaye & Lillyman (2000, p. 36) use the idea of 'reflection and a sense of soul' that feels appropriate to what has to be a focus of our work. They go on to write that:

> The view of reflective practice as being about 'self' opens up some interesting ideas. In everyday thinking, this is reflection aligned to self-study; it can help to make us more self-aware and self-conscious (in a positive way), and more in touch with the many sides of our personalities or multiple selves (Harre, 1998). It can be about self-esteem, self-concept and self-development. In healthcare we work with both head and heart. We must feelingly know what is the most appropriate way to care. We are not machines. We have feelings.
>
> When trying to develop reflective teams (and organisations) reflection-on-practice can help to provide a 'sense of soul to our work' [Hall, 1997]. It can help to bring everything together into a meaningful whole. (2000, p. 36)

They go on to state that this reflection on practice is based upon the following:

- Authenticity: coming to know our authentic self through meaningful relationships with others in our health-care team and organization.
- Intentionality: where our shared intentions are to act in a systematic, supportive, constructively critical and creative manner in order to enhance practice and the quality of care. This refers to putting our 'heart and soul' into realizing our hopes.
- Sensibility: reflective practitioners are sensitive to their own needs and wants and to the needs and wants of those they work with and care for; reflection heightens our sensitivities.
- Spirituality: reflection can foster a deep sense of obligation, commitment and moral purpose to our work. Through our caring practices, we appreciate a sense of connectedness and mutual interdependence with those for whom we care. Through reflection we experience a sense of being part of and connected to something larger and more significant than 'the self'. (2000, p. 36)

This development of a 'sense of soul' is a challenge to all of us as the case study presented in Chapter 9 makes only too clear. It may be worth revisiting that case study at this point.

> **Reflections**
>
> How does the evidence in the case study in Chapter 9 relate to what is set out above about reflection?

Having looked at the foundations upon which our practice is built and considered practical and theoretical issues relating to principles, the process of working and interacting with the group, the next ingredient to consider is the management and facilitation of sessions.

Management and facilitation of sessions

> In the first session I wondered what was going on at times you didn't seem to manage the group in the way I manage groups at work, but we did seem to start working together quickly.

Management sounds a strange word to be using within the context of human relations, as it immediately brings into play power relationships, the manager and the managed. The tutor in this setting needs to be a committed reflective practitioner with a strong understanding of the principle at the heart of reflective practice. The tutor needs to be able to allow the power relationships within the group to change. In describing the process of working, and in having considered the enabling environment, I have explored important aspects of facilitation in sessions.

I would now like to explore an important ingredient that is a thread in all of our work in this field and beyond in life in general. It is important in managing and facilitating enabling relationships. It is time.

Time – looking back to look forward

> What has been really useful, I know we have only had ten weeks, working together, is the way, although we've done a lot, look at the size of my portfolio, but there has always seemed to be time. We haven't rushed things.
>
> I didn't know how I came across when I communicated then but I do now.

It seems to me that this is one of the most powerful aspects of working with a group or, more fundamentally, a significant driver in our lives. Individuals will often say 'if I could only turn back time' or 'time is slipping away' or even 'time is a great healer'. We hear about it in daily conversation, in songs, read about it in books. The time 'slipping away' is a feeling I have as I write! Looking back and stopping time is a constant theme in our lives. Time is significant to us in so many ways. Salmon writes:

Seeing a snapshot of oneself at an earlier time can bring strong and complicated feelings. There we stand, confidently embedded in *that* present, entirely unaware of how old-fashioned, how quaint, we look. That is *us*, yet what an unbridgeable distance separates that person from the person living now! (1985, p. 12)

This is an important quote as it says so much about the experiences that individuals and groups feel and express in terms of their relationships with students, clients and colleagues. When we all stop and look back at those 'snapshots', we can often be surprised by what we see 'confidently embedded in *that* present'. 'I was unaware of how I interacted with my clients', 'I didn't know how I came across when I communicated then but I do now.' Salmon (1985) clearly expresses the idea that time is the key and has an important part to play in the process of reflection. This is about time to pause and to consider the narratives of our ways of being, and time, too, to reflect on these to see what we now have learnt, feel and understand.

Giving time and space to allow for this reflection and *looking back to look forward* is important. It allows for a growing sensitivity to develop both to our own needs and feelings, and to the needs and feelings of others.

I, therefore, hold to a strong belief that time is an important ingredient in the learning and teaching process, particularly in approaching enabling relationships. To be able to hold to the principles set out in Chapter 6 requires time on the part of the student and tutors. To be able to meet those principles, procedures and outcomes in this chapter requires time on the tutor's part. The overall experience and opportunities for both the learner and the tutor are affected by the time frame within which the course takes place. The spaces in between activities are as important as the activities themselves. Therefore, we have to ask ourselves if our work builds in sufficient time for opportunities to reflect. Does it give us suitable space to look back to consider what is meant by our central principle – to ensure that all those with whom we work are enabled to have a voice and to be able to share their thoughts, feelings and understandings about self and others through a mutually respectful dialogue? Is there time for a dialogue that is supported by unconditional positive regard that enables everyone to feel safe and valued as a person?

Like good pieces of music the silences are fundamental to making the sounds work as interesting textures to the ears. The spaces for *looking back to*

Reflections

Think about the nature of time in your work. What are the implications for structuring your sessions when viewed from a time perspective? What are the key points for you in relation to time? Write a statement about the nature of time and the work on enabling relationships that might go into a handbook on enabling relationships.

look forward are fundamental to making the actions work in the complex texture of enabling relationships.

The processes of working with a group on developing human relations are about enabling the individuals in the group to move forward on a journey. Our next question must therefore be:

WHAT KIND OF TUTOR IS NEEDED?

> I think that tutors have to be more in charge, well my team do at the college, otherwise the students wouldn't get anything done in time.

> You two are always very quiet in sessions with us aren't you? I don't mean you stay quiet, but you act in a quiet way, you listen and often somehow it feels as if all the ideas and thinking is ours!

In starting with the self in the developing and understanding of enabling relationships I think that it is important for us as tutors to start with ourselves. That is ourselves as individuals who will be managing, organizing and providing frameworks and structures for those in our groups. In developing your own reflective practice, it is worth reflecting on how you construe your role and the dilemmas inherent in that role for you. It is difficult to define the dilemmas that individual readers might have about the tutor's role in workshop sessions as I bring different experiences and expectations to the role.

In managing sessions in this area we have to remain true to allowing the process to develop strategies that can enable empowerment in those who form the group by assisting people to take greater control over their lives. Ashcroft & Foreman-Peck see this as 'a process of management of self and others' (1994, p. 1). This understanding is felt by us as individuals because it is more than conceptual development and change.

A PROGRAMME: TOWARDS FELT UNDERSTANDING

> Now I'm nearly at the end of the course, or journey as you keep calling it, I feel as if I understand the ideas not just in my head but as if it's real, which I know it is! Oh I can't explain it I just feel it.

> I know me in a different way as a practitioner.

Those who have journeyed with us through this book and shared and reflected on the ideas will know that the experience is not just a conceptual one, but a real and felt experience. A programme based on this book, therefore, explores people, their feelings, thoughts, identity, desires and the way that they communicate with each other.

This book can be a rich resource for the tutor who is developing a programme. Not, as I stated at the start of the chapter, as the recipe, but the ingredients. The chapters give you the theoretical material that can be used to enable your students to develop their own understanding of enabling relationships. This is an understanding grounded in rich material that we can use to inform ourselves, from which we can create our own sessions, or use the chapters as directed reading for students. The material requires of the students, and us, different forms of engagement and response through the reflections. This can also allow for individual, small-group or whole-group engagement and response, both within and outside sessions. In putting together your own programme, it is worth considering this balance.

The structuring and development of programmes of study in this field are not easy, particularly if you, as a tutor, hold reflective practice as the core of your work. If so, you will be committed to partnership in learning as well as in professional and clinical practice, with colleagues and client. In working you will be guided by principles for partnership and participation (see Chapter 6). I would suggest that the response to engaging in a programme, which explores these ideas, our feelings and understandings, creates a real impetus towards *felt understanding*, which, in turn, creates the basis for both integrated knowledge and truly reflective practice. It allows for the participants to bring to bear their knowledge of their real lived world to the sessions and activities within a programme. This approach can create a significant space and time for them as individuals, and in partnership with others in the group and the tutor, to *look back in order to look forward.*

CONCLUSION

I have tried to highlight the ingredients that need to be brought together to create opportunities for individuals and groups to reflect on enabling relationships. Through this process I hope to have helped individual tutors, through a sharpened sense of the issues involved in working with groups and individuals, to increase their potential to act adaptively in response to the needs and demands of those groups and individuals.

Remember it is our role to help our students to:

- enable themselves and others to have a voice and be heard
- respect the diversity of people's aspirations and values
- challenge the structural, attitudinal and environmental barriers that discriminate against ill and disabled people, women, ethnic groups and those with different expressions of gender.

It is your role to contribute to their development of what Postman & Weingartner call 'crap detectors' (1969, p. 16).

It is worth remembering at this point that through working with people we can be involved in opening doors to new ways of reflecting, thinking and being, but you cannot push someone through to a new or revised understanding. They have to want to make the journey.

> Thank God there are no free schools or printing. . . . For learning has brought disobedience and heresy into the world, and printing has divulged them. . . . God keep us from both. Governor of Virginia, d. 1677.

Acknowledgements: I am grateful to the students who have worked with me on a variety of courses that have looked at issues relating to human relationships and enabling relationships, and who have shared journeys into our own professional practice across a range of settings and professional groupings. I am also grateful to Helen Taylor for her time.

Still stumbling on: a conclusion

John Swain

I end where I began: stumbling on – still – to affirm a position in health and social care for therapists. To stumble on is to shift from the safe to the uncomfortable, from the assumed and accepted to the problematic and unknown, from answers to questions and from the certain to the uncertain. In her book on reflective practice for nurses, Taylor comes to a similar conclusion:

> Your biggest challenge will be to remain aware of the danger of familiarity and the tendency to accept a given reality as though it is as it should be and could be no other way. Life will be seen as 'work in progress' in which nothing is perfect or complete and everything can be seen afresh constantly to reveal new insights and possibilities for interpretation and adaptation. (2000, p. 245)

We have attempted to put critical reflection at the core of enabling relationships through and within therapy practice. It is a risky business. It is not simply about learning a set of predetermined skills to improve therapy, although interpersonal communication skills are clearly important. Let's conclude, then, by trying to pinpoint the key processes and sources of risk, uncertainty and questions.

Reflections

Looking back through your **REFLECTIONS**, what, for you, have been the critical moments, or critical incidents, that have enabled, opened, fuelled your reflections on, and development of, your practice in enabling relationships?
  I would point to a number of sources that I believe are pertinent whether within therapy practice, education or health and social care generally.

- The first has to be the expressed views of clients. Listening to clients is a major imperative in anything called 'enabling relationships'. But listening is also not enough. It is easy for professionals to listen for and hear the information they seek – in assessing and planning interventions. Enabling

(Continued)

Reflections — continued

relationships are fashioned between people in our interactions, understandings, purposes and desires – and in the shifting power relations between professionals and clients. Listening needs to be part of the building of partnerships and building working alliances with clients.

- Relationships can be enabled too through the stories participants tell and retell. The basis for empowerment can be in the insights afforded into motives, expectations, aims and convictions. Narratives can be grounded in the social processes, knowledge and self.
- Relationships are also contained, restrained, shaped, limited, given meaning – enabled and disabled – within the broader historical and social context that therapists and clients bring to therapy practice. Part of critically reflective practice has to be offering resources for criticizing established constructions of the social world and therapy practice itself, and unpacking their procedures for legitimization. This is an emphasis on the questioning of dominant ideologies, where social change is brought about through looking at and challenging the role of ideas and presumptions in legitimizing social relations and in not recognizing social divisions and even conflict.
- Perhaps the most intransigent barriers to enabling relationships are encompassed in the institutionalized discrimination that is built into the language that we use, the physical environment, the procedures, the rules, the lack of information in alternative formats, and the inflexible ways of working. Here is grist for the mill of critical reflection in the establishment of anti-discriminatory and anti-oppressive therapy practice – working in partnership and alliances with others.

So we who wrote this book together are still stumbling on – and that is a good place to be. We hope you have found it a good place to be too.

References

Abbott P 2000 Gender. In: Payne G (ed.) Social divisions. Macmillan Press, Houndmills

Abercrombie N, Hill S, Turner BS 1994 Dictionary of sociology, 3rd edn. Penguin, Harmondsworth

Aiello J, Douthitt E 2001 Social facilitation from Triplett to electronic performance monitoring. Group Dynamics 5(3): 163–180

Anderson H 1997 Conversation, language, and possibilities: a postmodern approach to therapy. BasicBooks, New York

Ashcroft K, Foreman-Peck L 1994 Managing teaching and learning in further and higher education. The Falmer Press, London

Aspen 1983 For my political sisters. In: The raving beauties in the pink. The Women's Press, London

Atkin K (In press) Health care for people from ethnic minority groups. In: French S, Sim J (eds.) Physiotherapy: a psychosocial approach, 3rd edn. Butterworth-Heinemann, Oxford

Atkinson D 1999 An old story. In: Swain J, French S (eds) Therapy and learning difficulties: advocacy, participation and partnership. Butterworth-Heinemann, Oxford

Atkinson D, Williams F (eds) 1990 'Know me as I am': an anthology of prose, poetry and art by people with learning difficulties. Hodder and Stoughton, Sevenoaks

Atkinson T, Claxton G 2000 The intuitive practitioners. Open University Press, London

Ball J, Norman A 2000 'Without the group, I'd still be eating half the co-op'. An example of groupwork with women who use food. Groupwork 9(1): 48–61

Banister P, Burman E, Parker I, Taylor M, Tindall C 1994 Qualitative methods in psychology: a research guide. Open University Press, Buckingham

Barnes C 1991 Disabled people in Britain and discrimination. Hurst & Co, London

Barnes M, Bowl R 2001 Taking over the asylum: empowerment and mental health. Palgrave, Houndmills

Barnitt R 2000 The virtuous therapist. In: Davies C, Finlay L, Bullman A (eds) Changing practice in health and social care. Sage in association with the Open University, London

Basnett I 2001 Health care professionals and their attitudes toward and decisions affecting disabled people. In: Albrecht G, Seelman K, Bury M (eds) Handbook of disability studies. Sage, London

Beauchamp TL, Childress JF 2001 Principles of biomedical ethics, 5th edn. Oxford University Press, Oxford

Becker G 1997 Disrupted lives: how people create meaning in a chaotic world. University of California Press, Berkeley & Los Angeles

Begum N 1994 Snow white. In: Keith L (ed.) Mustn't grumble: writing by disabled women. The Women's Press, London

Bender A, Ewashen C 2000 Group work is political work: a feminist perspective of interpersonal group psychotherapy. Issues in Mental Health Nursing 21(3): 297–308

Bennett P 1993 Counselling for heart disease. BPS Books, Leicester

Benzeval M, Judge K, Whitehead M 1995a Unfinished business. In: Benzeval M, Judge K, Whitehead M (eds) Tackling inequalities in health: an agenda for action. King's Fund, London

Benzeval M, Judge K, Whitehead M 1995b Introduction. In: Benzeval M, Judge K, Whitehead M (eds) Tackling inequalities in health: an agenda for action. King's Fund, London

Benzeval M, Judge K, Whitehead M 1995c The role of the NHS. In: Benzeval M, Judge K, Whitehead M (eds) Tackling inequalities in health: an agenda for action. King's Fund, London

Beresford P, Croft S, Evans C, Harding T 2000 Quality in personal social services: the developing role of user involvement in the UK. In: Davies C, Finlay L, Bullman A (eds) Changing practice in health and social care. Sage in association with the Open University, London

Berger P 1966 Invitation to sociology. Penguin, Harmondsworth

Biley FC 1992 Some determinants that affect patient participation in decision-making about nursing care. Journal of Advanced Nursing 17(4): 414–421

Blumer H 1989 Symbolic interactionism: perspective and method. Prentice Hall, London

Blumer H 1989 The Dilemma of Qualitative Measure. Routledge, London

Booth S, Swabey D 1999 Group training in communication skills for carers of adults with aphasia. International Journal of Language and Communication Disorders 34(3): 291–309

Bradley H 1996 Fractured identities: Changing patterns of inequality. Polity Press, Cambridge

Braham P, Janes L 2001 Social differences and divisions: introduction. In: Braham P, Janes L (eds) Social differences and divisions. Blackwell, Oxford

Braye S, Preston-Shoot M 1995 Empowering practice in social care. Open University Press, Buckingham

Brechin A 2000 Introducing critical practice. In: Brechin A, Brown H, Eby MA (eds) Critical practice in health and social care. Sage in association with the Open University, London

Brechin A, Swain J 1989 Creating a 'working alliance' with people with learning difficulties. In: Brechin A, Walmsley J (eds) Making connections: reflecting on the lives and experiences of people with learning difficulties. Hodder and Stoughton in association with the Open University, London

Brechin A, Brown H, Eby MA (eds) 2000 Critical practice in health and social care. Sage in association with the Open University, London

Brown F, Shiels M, Hall C 2001 A pilot community living skills group: an evaluation. British Journal of Occupational Therapy 64(3): 144–150

Brown H 1999 Finding out. Understanding health and social care. Open University Course (K100) Block 5, Unit 5. Open University, Milton Keynes

Brown H 2000 Challenges from service users. In: Brechin A, Brown H, Eby MA (eds) Critical practice in health and social care. Sage in association with the Open University, London

Brown JB, Weston WW 1995 Understanding the whole person. In: Stewart M, Brown JB, Weston WW, McWhinney IR, McWilliam CL, Freeman CR (eds) Patient-centred medicine: transforming the clinical method. Sage, London

Bruner J 1995 Meaning and self in cultural perspective. In: Bakhurst D, Sypnowich C (eds) The social self. Sage, London

Burnard P 1996 Acquiring interpersonal skills: a handbook of experiential learning for health professionals, 2nd edn. Stanley Thornes (Publishers) Ltd., Cheltenham

Burr V 1995 An introduction to social constructionism. Routledge, London

Butler J 1989 Gender trouble: feminism and the subversion of identity. Routledge, London

Cain P 2002 Cardiopulmonary resuscitation. In: Fulford KWM, Dickenson DL, Murray TH (eds) Healthcare ethics and human values: an introductory text with readings and case studies. Blackwell Publications, London

Cegala D, McClure L, Marinelli T, Post D 2000 The effects of communication skills training on patients' participation during medical interviews. Patient Education and Counselling 41(2): 209–222

Charmaz K 1991 Good days, bad days: the self in chronic illness and time. Rutgers University Press, New Brunswick, NJ

Chartered Society of Physiotherapy 1996 Rules of professional conduct. Physiotherapy 81: 460

Clarke C 2000 Professional ethics. In Davies M (ed.) The Blackwell encyclopaedia of social work. Blackwell Publishers, Oxford

Claxton G 2000 The Intuitive Practitioner: on the value of not always knowing what one is. Open University Press, Buckingham

Code C, Eales C, Pearl G, Conan M, Cowin K, Hickin J 2001 Profiling the membership of self-help groups for aphasic people. International Journal of Language and Communication Disorders 36: 41–45

Cole M 1998 Group dynamics in occupational therapy: the theoretical basis and practice application of group treatment. Slack, New Jersey

Constantino R, Bricker P 1996 Nursing postvention for spousal survivors of suicide. Issues in Mental Health Nursing 17(2): 131–152

Cooper M, Rowan J 1999 Introduction: self-plurality – the one and the many. In: Rowan J, Cooper M (eds) The plural self: multiplicity in everyday life. Sage, London

Corker M 1994 Counselling – the deaf challenge. Jessica Kingsley, London

Corker M 1996 Deaf transitions: images and origins of deaf families, deaf communities and deaf identities. Jessica Kingsley, London

Cousins SD 1989 Culture and self-perception in Japan and the United States. Journal of Personality and Social Psychology 56: 124–31

Crimmens P 1998 Storymaking and creative groupwork with older people. Jessica Kingsley, London

Crisp R 2002 A counselling framework for understanding individual experiences. Disability Studies Quarterly 22(3): 22–33

Crow L 1996 Including all of our lives: Renewing the social model of disability. In: Barnes C, Mercer G (eds) Exploring the divide: illness and disability. The Disability Press, Leeds

D'Aoust V 1996 Which map is not whose territory? In: Tremain S (ed.) Pushing the limits. Disabled dykes produce culture. The Women's Press, London

Dahlgren G, Whitehead M 1991 Policies and strategies to promote social equity in health. In: Benzeval M, Judge K, Whitehead M (eds) Tackling inequalities in health: an agenda for action. King's Fund, London

Dallos R 1997 Interacting stories: narratives, family beliefs and therapy. Karnac Books, London

Dalrymple J, Burke B 1995 Anti-oppressive practice: social care and the law. Open University Press, Buckingham

Davey B 1999 Solving economic, social and environmental problems together: an empowerment strategy for losers. In: Barnes M, Warren L (eds) Alliances and partnerships in empowerment. Polity Press, Bristol

Dekker K 1996 Why oblique and why Jung? In: Pearson J (ed.) Discovering the self through drama and movement. Jessica Kingsley, London

Demain S, Smith J, Hiller L, Dziedzic K 2001 Comparison of group and individual physiotherapy for female urinary incontinence in primary care: pilot study. Physiotherapy 87(5): 235–242

Department of Health 1999 Saving lives: our healthier nation. HMSO, London

Department of Health 2001 The national health inequalities targets. Department of Health, London

Department of Health, Social Services Inspectorate, Scottish Office, Social Work Services Group 1991 Care management and assessment: summary of practice guidance. HMSO/Scottish Office, Social Work Services Group, London

Dewey J 1933 How we think: a restatement of the relation of reflective thinking to the education process. Henry Regnery, Chicago

Dickson D, Hargie O, Morrow N 1997 Communication skills training for health professionals, 2nd edn. Chapman-Hall, London

Doel M, Sawdon C 1999 The essential groupworker: teaching and learning creative groupwork. Jessica Kingsley, London

Doktor D 1996 Dramatherapy and clients with eating disorders: fragile board. In: Mitchell S (ed.) Dramatherapy: clinical studies. Jessica Kingsley, London, pp. 179–193

Dominelli L 1997 Anti-racist social work, 2nd edn. Macmillan Press, Houndmills

Dominelli L 2002 Anti-oppressive social work theory and practice. Palgrave Macmillan, Houndmills

Donati S, Ward C 1999 Contexts for working in partnership. In: Swain J, French S (eds) Therapy and learning difficulties: advocacy, participation and partnership. Butterworth-Heinemann, Oxford

Drewery W, Winslade J 1997 The theoretical story of narrative therapy. In: Monk G, Winslade J, Crocket K, Epston D (eds) Narrative therapy in practice: the archaeology of hope. Jossey-Bass, San Francisco

Duggan C, Dijkers M 1999 Quality of life – peaks and valleys: a qualitative analysis of the narratives of persons with spinal cord injuries. Canadian Journal of Rehabilitation 12(3): 179–189

Eby MA 2000 The challenge of values and ethics in practice. In: Brechin A, Brown H, Eby MA (eds) Critical perspectives in health and social care. Sage in association with the Open University, London

Edge RS, Randall Groves J 1999 Ethics of health care: a guide for clinical practice, 2nd edn. Delmar Publishers, London

Edwards C 2002 A proposal that patients be considered honorary members of the healthcare team. Journal of Clinical Nursing 11(3): 340–348

Ellis-Hill C, Horn S 2000 Change in identity and self-concept: a new theoretical approach to recovery following a stroke. Clinical Rehabilitation 14(3): 279–287

Ellis-Hill C, Payne S, Ward C 2000 Self-body split: issues of identity in physical recovery following stroke. Disability and Rehabilitation 22(16): 725–733

Elman R, Bernstein-Ellis E 1999 The efficacy of group communication treatment in adults with chronic aphasia. Journal of Speech, Language and Hearing Research 42(2): 411–419

Finlay L 1997 Groupwork in occupational therapy. Nelson Thornes, Cheltenham

Finlay L 2000 The challenge of working in teams. In: Brechin A, Brown H, Eby MA (eds) Critical practice in health and social care. Sage, London

Firth P 2000 Picking up the pieces: groupwork in palliative care. Groupwork 12(1): 26–41

Fish D, Coles C 2000 Seeing anew: understanding professional practice as artistry. In: Davies C, Finlay L, Bullman A (eds) Changing practice in health and social care. Sage in association with the Open University, London

Foucault M 1982 An interview with Michel Foucault. In: Raus C (ed.) Death in the labyrinth: the world of Michel Foucault. Athlone Press, London

Fox J, Benzeval M 1995 Perspectives on social variations on health. Benzeval M, Judge K, Whitehead M (eds) Tackling inequalities in health: an agenda for action. King's Fund, London

Frank A 1995 The wounded storyteller: body, illness and ethics. University of Chicago Press, Chicago

Freedman J, Combs G 1996 Narrative therapy: the social construction of preferred realities. W. W. Norton and Company, New York

French S 1993 'Can you see the rainbow?' The roots of denial. In: Swain J, Finkelstein V, French S, Oliver M (eds) Disabling barriers – enabling environments. Sage, London

French S 1994 Attitudes of health professionals towards disabled people: a discussion and review of the literature. Physiotherapy 80: 687–693

French S 1997a Inequalities in health. In: French S (ed.) Physiotherapy: a psychosocial approach, 2nd edn. Butterworth-Heinemann, Oxford

French S 1997b Why do people become patients? In: French S (ed.) Physiotherapy: a psychosocial approach, 2nd edn. Butterworth-Heinemann, Oxford

French S 2001 Disabled people and employment: a study of the working lives of visually impaired physiotherapists. Ashgate, Aldershot

French S, Sim J 1993 Writing: a guide for therapists. Butterworth-Heinemann, Oxford

French S, Vernon A 1997 Health care for people from ethnic minority groups. In: French S (ed.) Physiotherapy: a psychosocial approach, 2nd edn. Butterworth-Heinemann, Oxford

French S, Swain J 2001 The relationship between disabled people and health and welfare professionals. In: Albrecht GL, Seelman KD, Bury M (eds) Handbook of disability studies. Sage, London

French S, Swain J 2002 Across the disability divide: whose tragedy? In: Fulford KWM, Dickenson DL, Murray TH (eds) Healthcare ethics and human values: an introductory text with readings and case studies. Blackwell Publications, London

Friere P 1972 Pedagogy of the oppressed. Penguin Books Ltd, London

Fuss D 1989 Essentially speaking: feminism, nature and difference. Routledge, London

Gambrill E 1990 Critical thinking in clinical practice. Jossey-Bass, San Francisco

Gelsomino K, Kirkpatrick L, Hess R, Gahimer J 2000 A descriptive analysis of physical therapy group intervention in five mid-western inpatient rehabilitation facilities. Journal of Physical Therapy Education 14(1): 12–20

Gergen KJ 1999 An invitation to social construction. Sage, London

Gerteis M, Edgman-Levitan S, Daley J, Delbanco T 1993 Medicine and health from the client's perspective. In: Gerteis M, Edgman-Levitan S, Daley J, Delbanco T (eds) Through the client's eyes: understanding and promoting client-centered care. Jossey-Bass, San Francisco

Getzel G, Mahoney K 1989 Confronting human finitude: groupwork with people with AIDS. Groupwork 2(2): 95–107

Ghaye A, Ghaye K 1998 Teaching and learning through critical reflective practice. David Fulton Publishers, London

Ghaye T, Lillyman S 2000 Reflection: principles and practice for healthcare professionals. Mark Allen Publishing Group, Dinton, Wiltshire

Giddens A 1991 Modernity and self-identity: self and society in the late modern age. Polity Press, Cambridge

Gillespie-Sells K, Campbell J 1991 Disability equality training: trainers guide. Central Council for Education and Training in Social Work, London

Gilligan C 1982 In a different voice: psychological development and women's moral development. Harvard University Press, Cambridge

Gilroy P 1997 Diaspora and the detours of identity. In: Woodward K (ed.) Identity and difference. Sage, London

Goffman E 1959 The presentation of self in everyday life. Doubleday, Garden City, NY

Gomm R 1993 Issues of power in health and welfare. In: Walmsley J, Reynolds J, Shakespeare P, Woolfe R (eds) Health, welfare and practice: reflecting on roles and relationships. Sage, London

Gough B, McFadden M 2001 Critical psychology: an introduction. Palgrave, Houndmills

Gould N 1996 Introduction: social work education and the 'crisis of the professions'. In: Gould N, Taylor I (eds) Reflective learning for social work. Arena, Aldershot

Graham-Pole J 2000 Illness and the art of creative self-expression. New Harbinger Publications, Oakland, CA

Gray A 2001 The decline of infectious diseases: the case of England. In: Gray A (ed.) World health and disease. Open University Press, Buckingham

Gray R, Fitch M, Phillips C, Labrecque M, Fergus K 2000 Managing the impact of illness: the experiences of men with prostate cancer and their spouses. Journal of Health Psychology 5(4): 531–548

Gross RD 2001 Psychology: the science of mind and behaviour, 4th edn. Hodder and Stoughton, London

Habermann U 1990 Self-help groups: a minefield for professionals. Groupwork 3(3): 221–235

Hall S 1990 Cultural identity and diaspora. In: Rutherford J (ed.) Identity: community, culture and difference. Lawrence and Wishart, London

Hall S 1997 Forms of reflective teaching practice in higher education. In: Pospisil R, Willcoxon L (eds) Learning through Teaching: 124–31. Proceedings of the 6th Annual Teaching Learning Forum, Murdoch University

Hallis M 1977 Models of man: philosophical thoughts on social action. Cambridge University Press, Cambridge

Hardy B 1968 Towards a poetics of fiction: an approach through narrative. Novel 2: 5–14

Harré R 1998 The Singular Self. An introduction to the psychology of personhood. Sage, London

Harre R, Gillett G 1994 The discursive mind. Sage, Thousand Oaks

Harrison T 1987 Selected poems, 2nd edn. Penguin Books, London

Hartley P 1999 Interpersonal communication, 2nd edn. Routledge, London

Hatt S 2000 The different worlds of work. In: Dawson G, Hatt S (eds) Market, state and feminism: the economics of feminist policy. Edward Elgar, Aldershot

Hayes N 2000 Foundations of psychology, 3rd edn. Thomson Learning, Albany, NY

helen (charles) (1993) 'Queer nigger': theorizing 'white' activism. In: Bristow J, Wilson AR (eds) Activating theory: lesbian, gay, bisexual politics. Lawrence and Wishart, London

Helitzer D, Cunningham-Sabo L, VanLeit B, Crowe T 2002 Perceived changes in self-image and coping strategies of mothers of children with disabilities. Occupational Therapy Journal of Research 22(1): 25–33

Hetherington K 1998 Expressions of identity: space, performance, politics. Sage, London

Hickey G, Kipping C 1998 Exploring the concept of user involvement in mental health through a participation continuum. Journal of Clinical Nursing 7(1): 83–88

Higgs R 1991 Looking after yourself. In: Corney R (ed.) Developing communication and counselling skills in medicine. Routledge, London

Hills J 1995 Joseph Rowntree Foundation inquiry into income and wealth, vols 1 and 2. Joseph Rowntree Foundation, York

HMSO (1996) Disability Discrimination Act. HMSO, London

Holliday-Willey L 1999 Pretending to be normal: living with Asperger's syndrome. Jessica Kingsley, London

Hollway W 1989 Subjectivity and method in psychology. Sage, London

Holman H, Lorig K 2000 Patients as partners in managing chronic disease: partnership is a prerequisite for effective and efficient health care. BMJ 320: 526–527

Homan R 1991 The Ethics of Social Research. Longman, London

Hughes G 1998 A suitable case for treatment? Constructions of disability. In: Saraga E (ed.) Embodying the social: constructions of difference. Routledge in association with the Open University, London

Hugman R 1991 Power in caring professions. Macmillan Press, Basingstoke

Hyde P 2001 Support groups for people who have experienced psychosis. British Journal of Occupational Therapy 64(4): 169–174

Iezzoni L 1998 What should I say? Communication around disability. Annals of Internal Medicine 129: 661–665

Israeli A, Santor D 2000 Reviewing effective components of feminist therapy. Counselling Psychology Quarterly 13(3): 233–247

James J 1996 Dramatherapy with people with learning disabilities. In: Mitchell S (ed.) Dramatherapy: clinical studies. Jessica Kingsley, London

Jenkins R 1996 Social identity. Routledge, London

Jennings C, Kennedy E (eds) 1996 The reflective professional in education: psychological perspectives on changing contexts. Jessica Kingsley, London

Johnson D, Johnson F 2002 Joining together: group theory and group skills. Allyn & Bacon, Needham Heights, MS

Jones L 2000 Behavioural and environmental influences on health. In: Katz J, Peberdy A, Douglas J (eds) Promoting health: knowledge and practice, 2nd edn. Palgrave, Basingstoke

Kasar J, Nelson Clark E 2000 Developing professional behaviors. Slack Incorporated, Thorofare, NJ

Kirklin D 2001 Creating space to reflect and connect. In: Kirklin D, Richardson R (eds). Medical humanities: a practical introduction. Royal College of Physicians, London

Kirschenbaum H, Henderson V 1990 The Carl Rogers reader. Constable, London

Kolb DA 1984 Experiential learning: experience as the source of learning and development. Practice-Hall, Englewood Cliffs

Kondo D 1990 Crafting selves: power, gender and discourses of identity in a Japanese Workplace. University of Chicago, Chicago

Lackner S, Goldenberg S, Arrizza G, Tjosvold I 1994 The contingency of social support. Qualitative Health Research 4(2): 224–243

Langan M 1998a The contested concept of 'need'. In: Langan M (ed.) Welfare: needs, rights and risks. Routledge, London

Langan M 1998b Rationing health care. In: Langan M (ed.) Welfare: needs, rights and risks. Routledge, London

Le Fanu J 1999 The rise and fall of modern medicine. Little, Brown and Company, London

Leon D, Walt G 2001 Poverty, inequality and health in international perspective: a divided world? In: Leon D, Walt G (eds) Poverty, inequality and health: an international perspective. Oxford University Press, Oxford

Leventhal H, Idler E, Leventhal E 1999 The impact of chronic illness on the self system. In: Contrada R, Ashmore R, (eds) Self, social identity & physical health. Oxford University Press, Oxford, pp. 185–208

Ley P 1988 Communicating with clients. Chapman & Hall, London

Lillyman S 2000 Critical incidents as caring moments. In: Ghaye T, Lillyman S (eds) Caring moments: the discourse of reflective practice. Mark Allen Publishing Group, Salisbury

Lindesmith AR 1999 Symbolic interactionism. In: Lindesmith AR, Strauss AL, Denzin NK. Social psychology, 8th edn. Sage Publications, London

Lorde A 1984 Sister outsider: essays and speeches. The Crossing Press/Freedom, CA

Mackintosh M, Mooney G 2000 Identity, inequality and social class. In: Woodward K (ed.) Questioning identity: gender, class, nation. Routledge in association with the Open University, London

Madison GB 1988 The hermeneutics of postmodernity. Indiana University Press, Bloomington

Marks D 1999 Disability: controversial debates and psychosocial perspectives. Routledge, London

Marks D 2002 Introduction: counselling, therapy and emancipatory praxis. Disability Studies Quarterly 22(3): 2–6

Martin B 1988 Lesbian identity and autobiographical difference(s). In: Brodzki B, Shenck C (eds) Life/lines. Theorising women's autobiography. Cornell University Press, Ithaca, NY

Martin E, Ramsden P 1987 Learning skills, or skill in learning? In: Richardson JTE, Eysenck MW, Warren Piper D (eds) Student learning: research in education and cognitive psychology. Oxford University Press, Oxford

Mason M 2000 Incurably human. Working Press, London

Mason M, Rieser R 1992 The limits of 'medicine'. In: Rieser R, Mason M (eds) Disability equality in the classroom: a human rights issue. Disability Equality in Education, London

Mason S 2000 Groupwork with schizophrenia: clinical aspects. Groupwork 12(2): 27–44

Mason-John V, Khambatta A 1993 Lesbians talk. Making Black Waves. Scarlet Press, London

Mathieson C, Stam H 1995 Renegotiating identity: cancer narratives. Sociology of Health & Illness 17(3): 283–306

Mathiowitz V, Matuska K, Murphy M 2001 Efficacy of an energy conservation course for persons with multiple sclerosis. Archives of Physical Medicine and Rehabilitation 82(4): 449–456

Mattingly C 1998 Healing dramas and clinical plots: the narrative structure of experience. Cambridge University Press, Cambridge

McGraw M 1999 Studio-based art therapy for medically ill and physically disabled persons. In: Malchiodi C (ed.) Medical art therapy with adults. Jessica Kingsley, London, pp. 243–262

McKeown T 1984 The medical contribution. In: Black N, Boswell D, Gray A, Murphy S, Popay J (eds) Health and disease: a reader. Open University Press, Buckingham

McLeod J 1998a An introduction to counselling, 2nd edn. Open University Press, Buckingham

McLeod J 1998b Listening to stories about illness and health: applying the lessons of narrative psychology. In: Bagne R, Nicolson R, Horton I (eds) Counselling and communication skills for medical and health practitioners. British Psychological Society, Leicester

McWilliam C, Stewart M, Brown J, Desai K, Coderre P 1996 Creating health with chronic illness. Advances in Nursing Science 18(3): 1–15

Mercer G, Barnes C 2000 Disability: from medical needs to social rights. In: Tovey P (ed.) Contemporary primary care: the challenges for change. Open University Press, Buckingham

Miller C, Freeman M, Ross N 2001 Interprofessional practice in health and social care: challenging the shared learning agenda. Arnold, London

Milner J 2001 Women and social work: narrative approaches. Palgrave, Houndmills

Minar V 1999 Art therapy and cancer: images of the hurter and healer. In: Malchiodi C (ed.) Medical art therapy with adults. Jessica Kingsley, London

Molloy H, Vasil L 2002 The social construction of Asperger syndrome: the pathologising of difference? Disability & Society 17(6): 659–669

Monks J 1999 'It works both ways': belonging and social participation among women with disabilities. In: Yuval-Davis N, Werbner P (eds) Women, citizenship and difference. Zed Books, London

Morris D 2001 A few thoughts on independent living and taking control for the first time. In: Vasey S (ed.) The rough guide to managing personal assistants. National Centre for Independent Living, London

Morris J 1991 Pride against prejudice. The Women's Press, London

Munson R 1996 Intervention and reflection: basic issues in medical ethics, 5th edn. Wadsworth Publications Co, Belmont, CA

Nias J (ed.) The enquiring teacher: supporting and sustaining teacher research. Falmer Press, London

Nichols K 1989 Institutional versus client-centred care in general hospitals. In: Broome A (ed.) Health psychology: processes and applications. Chapman & Hall, London, pp. 103–113

Nightingale DJ, Cromby J 1999 Social constructionist psychology: a critical analysis of theory and practice. Open University Press, Buckingham

Nosko A, Breton M 1997–8 Applying a strength, competence and empowerment model. Groupwork 10(1): 55–69

Nylund M 2000 The mixed-based nature of self-help groups in Finland. Groupwork 12(2): 64–85

Oliver M 1990 The politics of disablement. Macmillan Press, Houndmills

Oliver M 1998 Theories in health care and research: theories of disability in health practice and research. BMJ 317(7170): 1446–1449

Oliver M, Barnes C 1998 Disabled people and social policy: from exclusion to inclusion. Longman, London

Ouimet M, Primeau F, Cole M 2001 Psychosocial risk factors in post-stroke depression: a systematic review. Canadian Journal of Psychiatry 46(9): 819–828

Øvretveit J, Mathias P, Thompson T (eds) 1997 Interprofessional working for health and social care. Macmillan, Basingstoke

Pahl R 1995 Cited in Clarke J (1998) Consumerism. In: Hughes G (ed.) Imagining welfare futures. Routledge, London

Paterson K, Hughes B 1999 Disability Studies and phenomenology: the carnal politics of everyday life. Disability & Society 14(5): 597–610

Payne G 2000 An introduction to social division. In: Payne G (ed.) Social divisions. Macmillan Press, Houndmills

Pearce WB 1994 Interpersonal communication: making social worlds. HarperCollins College, New York

Pearson J 1996 Discovering the self. In: Pearson J (ed.) Discovering the self through drama and movement. Jessica Kingsley, London

Penttinen J, Nevala-Puranen N, Airaksinen O et al. 2002 Randomised controlled trial of back school with and without peer support. Journal of Occupational Rehabilitation 12(1): 21–29

Peters S 1999 Transforming disability identity through critical literacy and the cultural politics of language. In: Corker M, French S (eds) Disability discourse. Open University Press, Buckingham

Piccirillo E 1999 Beyond words: the art of living with AIDS. In: Malchiodi C (ed) Medical art therapy with adults Jessica Kingsley Publishers, London

Postman N, Weingartner C 1969 Teaching as a subversive activity. Penguin Educational, London

Potter J 1998 Fragments in the realization of relativism. In: Parker I (ed.) Social constructionism, discourse and realism. Sage, London

Poulton B 1999 User involvement in identifying health needs and shaping and evaluating services: is it being realised? Journal of Advanced Nursing 30(6): 1289–1296

Pound C (In press) Dare to be different the person and the practice. In: Byng S, Duchan J (In press) Challenging therapies. Psychology Press, Hove

Predeger E 1996 Womanspirit: a journey into healing through art in breast cancer. Advances in Nursing Science 18(3): 48–58

Priestley M 1999 Disability politics and community care. Jessica Kingsley, London

Prior S 1998 Determining the effectiveness of a short-term anxiety management course. British Journal of Occupational Therapy 61(5): 207–213

Read S, Papakosta-Harvey V, Bower S 2000 Using workshops on loss for adult with learning disabilities. Groupwork 122: 6–26

Reimers S, Treacher A 1995 Introducing user-friendly family therapy. Routledge, London

Reynolds F 1999a When models of health care collide: a qualitative study of rehabilitation counsellors' reflections on working in physical health care settings. Journal of Interprofessional Care 13(4): 367–379

Reynolds F 1999b Creative arts activities and therapies. In: Swain J, French S (eds) Therapy and learning difficulties. Butterworth-Heinemann, Oxford

Reynolds S, Trinder L 2000 Evidence-based practice: a critical approach. Blackwell Science, Oxford

Riley S 2001 Group process made visible: group art therapy. Brunner-Routledge, Philadelphia

Ringer TM 2002 Group action: the dynamics of groups in therapeutic, educational and corporate settings. Jessica Kingsley, London

Rishty A 2000 The strengths perspective in reminiscence groupwork with depressed older adults. Groupwork 12(3): 37–55

Roberts J 1995 Group psychotherapy. British Journal of Psychiatry 166(1): 124–129

Robinson M 2002 Communication and health in a multi-ethnic society. The Policy Press, Bristol

Rogers C 1967 On becoming a person. Constable, London

Rogers C 1986 A client-centred/person-centred approach to therapy. In: Kutash I, Wolf A (eds) Psychotherapist's casebook. Jossey-Bass, New York

Rogers WA 2002 Evidence-based medicine in practice: limiting or facilitating patient choice? Health Expectations 5(2): 95–103

Ross W, Hannay L 1986 Towards a critical theory of reflective. Journal of Teacher Education XXXVII(4): 9–15

Rowland S 1993 The enquiring tutor. Falmer Press, London

Rumbold C 2000 Ethics in nursing practice. Bailliere Tindall, London

Rungapadiachy DV 1999 Interpersonal communication and psychology for health care professionals: theory and practice. Butterworth-Heinemann, Oxford

Saljo R 1979 Learning in the Learner's Perspective 1-Some Common sense Conceptions in Reports from the Institute of Education, University of Gothenberg, No. 77. Cited in Martin E, Ramsden P 1987 Learning skills or skills in learning. In: Student Learning: research in education and cognitive psychology. Richardson JTE et al 1987, OUP

Salmon 1980 Introduction to Coming to know. Salmon P (ed) Routledge & Kegan Paul Ltd, London

Salmon P 1985 Living in time. J.M. Dent and Sons, London

Saraga E 1998 Review. In: Saraga E (ed.) Embodying the social: constructions of difference. Routledge in association with the Open University, London

Schaverian J 1991 The revealing image: analytical art psychotherapy in theory and practice. Tavistock/Routledge, London

Schön D 1983 The reflective practitioner: how professionals think in action. Basic Books, New York

Schön D 1987 Educating the reflective practitioner: towards a new design for teaching and learning in the professions. Jossey-Bass, San Francisco, CA

Schwartz C, Sendor M 1999 Helping others helps oneself: response shift effects in peer support. Social Science & Medicine 48(11): 1563–1575

Schwartz L, Kraft G 1999 The role of spouse responses to disability and family environment in multiple sclerosis. American Journal of Physical Medicine and Rehabilitation 78(6): 525–532

Serlin I, Classen C, Frances B, Angell K 2000 Support groups for women with breast cancer: Traditional and alternative expressive approaches. Arts in Psychotherapy 27(2): 123–138

Seymour W 1998 Remaking the body: rehabilitation and change. Routledge, London

Shaughnessy P, Cruse S 2001 Health promotion with people who have a learning disability. In: Thompson J, Pickering S (eds) Meeting the health needs of people who have a learning disability. Bailliere Tindal, London

Sherwin S 2002 Towards a feminist ethics of health care. In: Fulford KWM, Dickenson DL, Murray TH (eds) Healthcare ethics and human values: an introductory text with readings and case studies. Blackwell Publications, London

Sim J 1997a Ethical decision making in therapy practice. Butterworth-Heinemann, Oxford

Sim J 1997b Ethics and moral decision making. In: French S (ed.) Physiotherapy: a psychosocial approach. Butterworth-Heinemann, Oxford

Smith SK 2000 Sensitive issues in life story research. In: Moch SD, Gates MF (eds) The researcher experience in qualitative research. Sage, Thousand Oaks

Somers M 1994 The narrative construction of identity: a relational and network approach. Theory and Society 23: 606–649

Souza A, Ramcharan P 2001 Being well and my well-being. In: Thompson J, Pickering S (eds) Meeting the health needs of people who have a learning disability. Bailliere Tindal, London

Standing S 1999 The practice of working in partnership. In: Swain J, French S (eds) Therapy and learning difficulties: advocacy, participation and partnership. Butterworth-Heinemann, Oxford

Steiner M 1992 Alternatives in psychiatry: dance movement therapy in the community. In: Payne H (ed.) Dance movement therapy: theory and practice. Routledge, London

Stevenson O, Parsloe P 1993 Community care and empowerment. Joseph Rowntree Foundation, York

Stewart M, Brown J B, Weston W W et al (eds). 1995 Patient-centreed medicine: Transforming the clinical method. Sage, London

Stuifbergen A, Rogers S 1997 Health promotion: an essential component of rehabilitation for persons with chronic disabling conditions. Advances in Nursing Science 19(4): 1–20

Sumsion T, Craik C, Glossop J 1999 Client-centred practice in occupational therapy. Churchill-Livingstone, London

Sutherland A 1981 Disabled we stand. Souvenir Press, London

Swain J 1995 The use of counselling skills: a guide for therapists. Butterworth-Heinemann, Oxford

Swain J, Lawrence P 1994 Learning about disability: changing attitudes or challenging understanding? In: French S (ed.) On equal terms: working with disabled people. Butterworth-Heinemann, Oxford

Swain J, Gillman M, French S 1998 Confronting disabling barriers: towards making organisations accessible. Venture Press, Birmingham

Swain J, Cameron C 1999 Unless otherwise stated: discourses of labelling and identity in coming out. In: Corker M, French S (eds) Disability discourse. Open University Press, Buckingham

Swain J, French S 2000 Towards an affirmative model of disability. Disability and Society 15(4): 569–582

Swain J, French S, Cameron C 2003 Controversial issues in a disabling society. Open University Press, Buckingham

Taskinen P 1999 The development of health enhancing exercise groups adapted for hemiplegic patients: a pilot study. Neurorehabilitation 13(1): 35–43

Taylor BJ 2000 Reflective practice: a guide for nurses and midwives. Open University Press, Buckingham

Thomas C 1999 Narrative identity and the disabled self. In: Corker M, French S (eds) Disability discourse. Open University Press, Buckingham

Thompson J, Pickering S (eds) 2001 Meeting the health needs of people who have a learning disability. Bailliere Tindal, London

Thompson N 1993 Anti-discriminatory practice, 2nd edn. Macmillan Press, London

Thompson N 1998 Promoting equality. Macmillan Press, London

Thompson N 2000 Theory and practice in human services. Open University Press, Buckingham

Thompson N 2001 Anti-Discriminatory practice, 3rd edn. Palgrave, Houndmills

Thompson S, Kyle D 2000 The role of perceived control in coping with the losses associated with chronic illness. In: Harvey J, Miller E (eds) Loss and trauma: general and close relationship perspectives. Brunner-Routledge, Philadelphia, pp. 131–145

Tierney S 2002 Anorexia: illuminating impairment of dishonourable disability? Disability Studies Quarterly 22(3): 6–21

Townsend E, Birch D, Langley J, Langille L 2000 Participatory research in a mental health clubhouse. Occupational Journal of Research 20(1): 18–44

Trnobranski P 1994 Nurse–patient negotiation: assumption or reality. Journal of Advanced Nursing 19: 733–737

Tudor Hart J 1971 The Inverse Care Law. The Lancet 1: 405–412

Union of the Physically Impaired Against Segregation 1976 Fundamental principles of disability. UPIAS, London

United Nations 1993 Standard Rules on the Equalization of Opportunities for People with Disabilities. General Assembly, Resolution 48/96, 20th December 1993

VanderVoort L, Duck S 2000 Talking about 'relationships': variations on a theme. In: Dindia K, Duck S (eds) Communication and personal relationships. John Wiley, Chichester

Vernon A, Swain J 2002 Theorizing divisions and hierarchies: towards a commonality or diversity? In: Barnes C, Oliver M, Barton L (eds) Disability Studies Today. Polity, Cambridge

Weber M 1978 Economy and Society Vols 1 & 2 (edited by Roth G & Wittich C) University of California Press, Berkley

Weitzenkamp D, Gerhart K, Charlifue S, et al. 2000 Ranking the criteria for assessing quality of life after disability: evidence for priority shifting among long-term spinal cord injury survivors. British Journal of Health Psychology 5(1): 57–70

Wendell S 1996 The rejected body: feminist philosophical perspectives on disability. Routledge, London

Wetherell M, Maybin J 1996 The distributed self: a social constructionist perspective. In: Stevens R (ed.) Understanding the self. Sage, London

Whitehead M 1995 Tackling inequalities: a review of policy initiatives. In: Benzeval M, Judge K, Whitehead M (eds) Tackling inequalities in health: an agenda for action. King's Fund, London

Widdershoven GAM 1993 The story of life: hermeneutic perspectives on the relationships between narrative and history. In: Josselson R, Lieblich A (eds) The narrative story of lives. Sage, Thousand Oaks

Widdershoven GAM, Smits M-J 1996 Ethics and narratives. In: Josselson R, Lieblich A (eds) The narrative story of lives. Sage, Thousand Oaks

Wilkinson S 1988 The role of reflexivity in feminist psychology. Women's Studies International Forum 11: 493–502

Williams F 1996 Postmodernism, feminism and the question of difference. In: Parton N (ed.) Social theory, social change and social work. Routledge, London

Williams G 2001 Theorizing disability. In: Albrecht G, Seelman K, Bury M (eds) Handbook of disability studies. Sage, Thousand Oaks

Wilson A and Beresford P 2000 Anti-oppressive practice: emancipation and appropriation British Journal of Social Work 30 553–73

Wilson J (1999) Acknowledging the expertise of patients and their organisations. BMJ, 18 September, 771–774

Woodward K 2000 Questions of identity. In: Woodward K (ed.) Questioning identity: gender, class, nation Routledge in association with the Open University, London

Worden JW 1983 Grief counselling and grief therapy. Tavistock Publications, London

Yalom I 1985 The theory and practice of group psychotherapy. Basic Books, New York

Index